The Art of Health Hacking is simply a game-changer. TJ doesn't just talk the talk—he walks the walk of optimal, holistic health. His creative, self-coach approach will inspire you to see your health as a hobby and guide you to building a deeper, more loving, and care-filled relationship with your Self and others. If you want to elevate your state of health and performance and have fun doing it, trust me—you must read this book.

JJ VIRGIN, CNS
4X *NEW YORK TIMES* BEST SELLING AUTHOR, *THE VIRGIN DIET*

Read *The Art of Health Hacking* to learn how vulnerability, self-compassion, and personal health empowerment can put you back in charge of yourself. TJ shows us we don't lack the science or technology to live healthy, but the art to use these resources properly. If you're on a path to better health, but are still looking to take it to the next level, then grab a copy of this book. You'll be glad you did.

DAVE ASPREY, FOUNDER OF BULLETPROOF
NEW YORK TIMES BEST SELLING SCIENCE AUTHOR, *HEAD STRONG*

TJ is a model for the health hacker of the future. Through his own health hacking adventures, *The Art of Health Hacking* tells the story of what's possible in our world today when it comes to biohacking your body and optimizing your health. TJ also shows it's not just about mastering your health, but how you can grow closer to yourself, God, and others. If you want to live with less stress, better relationships, and more resilient health, then you're going to dig this book.

BEN GREENFIELD, NSCA, ISSN
AUTHOR OF *NEW YORK TIMES* BESTSELLER, *BEYOND TRAINING*,
AND THE *CHRISTIAN GRATITUDE JOURNAL*

T0098600

TJ has brought his unbridled enthusiasm for life and optimal health into play in *The Art of Health Hacking*. The sparkplug ideas he shares in this book underscore his life-lived understanding that one's health status is preponderantly a reflection of chosen personal behaviors and accountability. If you desire becoming architect of your own bright health future, his lessons and suggested health hacks are a great place to start that journey.

WILLIAM K. APPELGATE, PHD, CPC
PRESIDENT AND FOUNDER OF THE CLINICAL HEALTH COACH®

The Art of Health Hacking is one of the best modern-day health guides I've seen. Through his unique self-coach approach, TJ provides an empowering way for patients to take advantage of the true healing available. As a doctor, seeing patients take responsibility for their health is both inspiring and necessary. No matter where you're at on the health spectrum, this book can help you put into practice the habits and routines necessary to achieve the health you desire.

KATHERINE ZAGONE, NATUROPATHIC DOCTOR
FOUNDER OF THE HOLISTIC FERTILITY METHOD

TJ has written one of the most comprehensive books on optimal health and sustainable behavior change I've ever seen. From blood work to breath work and everything in between, *The Art of Health Hacking* will guide you to becoming a healthier, powerful, and more loving version of yourself. If you want the ultimate book to self-coach your way to optimized health, this book has your name written all over it.

TONY STUBBLEBINE
CHIEF COACH, COACH.ME

The Art of Health Hacking

The Art of Health Hacking

THE 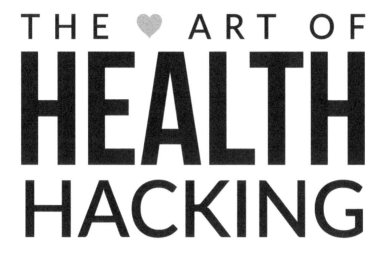 ART OF
HEALTH
HACKING

A Personal Guide to **Elevate Your State** of Health and Performance, Stress Less, and Build Healthy Habits that Matter

TJ ANDERSON

NEW YORK

LONDON • NASHVILLE • MELBOURNE • VANCOUVER

The Art of Health Hacking

A Personal Guide to Elevate Your State of Health and Performance, Stress Less, and Build Healthy Habits that Matter

Published in New York, New York, by Morgan James Publishing. Morgan James is a trademark of Morgan James, LLC. www.MorganJamesPublishing.com

The Morgan James Speakers Group can bring authors to your live event. For more information or to book an event visit The Morgan James Speakers Group at www.TheMorganJamesSpeakersGroup.com.

ISBN 9781683507734 paperback
ISBN 9781683507758 case laminate
ISBN 9781683507741 eBook
Library of Congress Control Number: 2017914682

Cover Design by:
Rachel Lopez
www.r2cdesign.com

Interior Design by:
Chris Treccani
www.3dogcreative.net

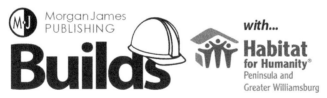

In an effort to support local communities, raise awareness and funds, Morgan James Publishing donates a percentage of all book sales for the life of each book to Habitat for Humanity Peninsula and Greater Williamsburg.

Get involved today! Visit
www.MorganJamesBuilds.com

DEDICATION

This book is dedicated to two of the most loving, hard-working entrepreneurs in this world—my parents.

A portion of author royalties will be donated to the Garden For Every School Project (http://www.gardens.school), which provides free, comprehensive video training and resources for K-12 school teachers and students to start and maintain a school garden.

CONTENTS

FOREWORD

---

by Dr. Anthony Balduzzi

We are living in one of the most pivotal times in human history.

Millions of us are hanging from a cliff—clinging for dear life as dirt slides beneath our fingernails. We're being dragged further down by the excess weight, stress, and disease of modern living. And what happens next will determine how this story ends.

The hard truth is that so many of us are not struggling with our health because of a **lack of information** about what we "should" be doing with our eating and exercise. There are more diet books, pills, blogs, and exercise gadgets than at any other time in human history.

So many of us are struggling because we lack something deeper: a process that enables us to heal our bodies, nourish our minds, and gently guide ourselves to greater health for the long haul.

My name is Dr. Anthony Balduzzi, and I am a health hacker. Over the past two decades, I've dedicated my life to the sole mission of helping pull people up off the cliff.

From a very young age, I learned the importance of health after watching my own father work himself to the bone, get sick, and pass away at forty-two years young. Through my work as the founder of The Fit Father Project, I've had the privilege of watching tens of thousands of men and their families improve their health and transform their lives.

I've seen what works and what doesn't. And this special book uncovers how you and I can pull **ourselves and those we love** up off the cliff once and for all. That's my and TJ's promise to you. Welcome to *The Art of Health Hacking.*

I don't know of anyone else who could have written this book besides Thomas Joel Anderson. In a way, this book is his calling—the perfect culmination of a set of diverse and seemingly disconnected life experiences that have come together to form a masterpiece.

That's what you're holding in your hands right now—a proven system that will empower you to reach your ideal level of health and maintain it for life.

See, TJ is so much more than your run-of-the-mill health expert, doctor, or personal trainer. He's the rare kind of person who still has pure childhood curiosity. He hasn't been tainted by too many detached medical journals, facts, and figures. If you've met TJ, then you know what I'm talking about. If you haven't, then you're definitely in for a treat.

Yet, it's not just his passionate, caring heart that makes TJ so special. It's his laser-sharp intellect and inspiring vulnerability that makes him particularly suited to share this message of empowered health with the world.

I've been studying health, medicine, and peak human performance for over two decades now. I can firmly say that TJ has taught me more valuable lessons through the principles in this book than years of intensive study have brought me.

That's why I'm so excited for you right now. You're about to discover these life-changing lessons and how you can apply them to reach greater levels of health and happiness.

See, there's an art and process to creating and maintaining health. It's a path that's both structured and fluid. By walking this path, you'll discover how to coach yourself to greater levels of health, energy, fitness, and joy—while also inspiring all those around you to do the same.

I'm writing this foreword because I deeply believe in this work.

To be completely honest, I would have turned down the opportunity to write the foreword for another potential best-selling, fad diet book that promises the next miracle, "quick fix" diet to cure all health problems forever. From seeing the last dozen of those books come and go from the shelves, you and I both know that information will be outdated and contradicted within a year.

The Art of Health Hacking is something radically different, and the principles contained herein **will stand the test of time**. I don't confidently say that simply because the health information in this book is incredibly sound. It certainly is. TJ has spent the past three years traveling around the world interviewing top experts in the fields of nutrigenomics, the science of behavioral change, and functional medicine.

Yet, it's not the proven science that makes this book special. I can confidently say this book will stand the test of time, because it's really a book about art. It's a book about how you and I can manage and enhance our health—amidst the busyness of life—in ways that go far beyond the calories, grams, facts, and figures.

TJ will help you uncover the missing piece you've been searching for: a system for both building the lean, energetic, flexible body you've always wanted—while also finding more self-compassion and appreciation for the process. This book will certainly help with that, but it's not *just* a book for us. This book is also for our children and their children too. They will follow our lead and learn from our example. This book will guide them in the right direction.

Welcome to *The Art of Health Hacking*, my friend. May you live long, live happy, and prosper.

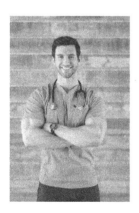

Dr. Anthony Balduzzi

Dr. Anthony Balduzzi
Naturopath Medical Doctor
CEO, Peak Performance Rx
Founder, Fit Father Project
*Has helped over 10,000 fathers
lose over 75,000 lbs of fat*

NOTE TO THE READER

Encinitas, California
February 6, 2017

When my ulnar nerve glides in and out of my right elbow socket, I don't say, "Oh, my funny bone!" and start to laugh in surprise. This sensation is different. And not funny at all.

Instead, I ask myself…

"Why the hell am I doing this?"

"Why did I write a book about hacking my health when the very act of writing (i.e., typing on a keyboard) is leading to the most annoying pain and discomfort in my hand, arm, and wrist?!"

Add a right hip issue, C5-C6 bulged disc, occasional symptoms of Temporomandibular Joint Disorder (a.k.a. TMJ/TMD), and tendonitis in my right forearm (probably from overusing the spectacular—yet at times soul-sucking—black-mirrored piece of technology in my pocket), and you'll have a partial list of the key "issues in my tissues" I'm consciously working on. But don't worry, I'm preventing cancer by blocking the radiation from my phone with an anti-radiation phone case designed by SafeSleeve, a company based out of San Diego.

Hey, I'm TJ.

And for the past seven years, I've been working at the intersection of health care and self-care. I've served as a health coach and health care consultant, but I've also been a "health hacker," optimizing my own health in the process. Let's

just say I've learned a thing or two about what *to do* and what *not to do* when it comes to coaching oneself to better health. As the subtitle suggests, I'm here to help you elevate your state of health and performance. **I'm not a doctor. But I am a trained health coach and self-taught self coach who knows a thing or two about sustainable health improvement.**

I've become the CEO of my own health care and self-care strategy. And now I'm here to help others, perhaps even you, do the same.

Over the past seven years, I've served as a health coach for entrepreneurs, a Group Fitness Instructor, as well as a health consultant for large hospitals, medical groups, community health centers, and physical therapy companies across the United States. But in the past three or four years, I've also ventured down an alternative path—the path of self-experimentation and self-research into my own health—holistically.

You see, we all have our own past experiences with health, wellness, fitness, and the entire health care system. And we're all currently at a different point on the health spectrum. But knowing where we stand in our health today and where we want to go requires a new, modern-day, self-coach approach.

The intention isn't to be perfect. I have my fair share of annoying health issues going on, and you may as well.

The key intention is to develop our awareness, listen, and tap into our intuition so we can learn how to ask ourselves the right questions.

And when we're ready, know where we feel called to act and experiment with new approaches to our health.

Here are a few questions for you to ponder…

- Do you know **where you are** (currently) in your health?
- Do you know **where you want to go**?
- Do you sometimes feel overwhelmed with charting the best possible course to **disease prevention** and **health optimization**?
- Have you taken action to **surround yourself** with other health-conscious consumers? Have you **supported others** in their own health journey as well?
- And, perhaps most importantly, do you know the **potential health blind spots** and **limiting beliefs** that might be holding you back?

Now, you might be wondering what I mean when I refer to myself as a "health hacker." We'll dive deeper into this term later, but for the record, we won't be stealing anyone's information in this book. Rather, we'll be igniting a new level of personal health empowerment, where we can all choose the state of health we want to create. We all have the power to take our overall health, energy, and life performance to another level—sometimes we just need to get a bit more creative.

So what is this book, *The Art of Health Hacking,* all about?

The subtitle explains what you can expect from this book. It truly is: **A Personal Guide to Elevate Your State of Health and Performance, Stress Less, and Build Healthy Habits that Matter.**

It's not just about taking your health to a new level, it's also about connecting the dots between your health and how you perform in your work and relationships. We will examine our relationship with stress, and, perhaps most importantly, we will dive into the process of building healthy habits that matter—the behaviors and actions that will make a profound difference in your life.

Note: I'm not writing this book simply as an expert **telling** you what you should do, either. Rather, I'm sharing what I've learned in my own life, both as a health coach and a self coach, in my quest toward living a healthy, happy, disease-free life. May this book act as your **personal guide.** And may whatever is meant to unfold, unfold.

Why the "Art" of Health Hacking?

The science and technology are here, my friends. Those are not what we lack to prevent disease and live healthy. We need to develop the *art* of marrying the science and theoretical concepts with action, so we can apply what we've learned and actually see noticeable results. The red heart at the top of this book's cover was included for a reason.

We must also cultivate the *heart* to develop deeper relationships with ourselves and others. If we want to make more health-conscious, intentional choices in each and every new moment, we need to infuse more heart.

When we create harmony in our health, we develop the capacity to become not simply health experts, but self experts.

WE DON'T LACK THE HEALTH EXPERTS.
WE LACK THE SELF EXPERTS.

What exactly do I mean by this?

Well, just think about it.

Are we missing more health experts—people who know a lot about health? Or are we missing more *self experts*—people who know how to take care of themselves?

In my experience, there are a lot of people who have general health knowledge—like the importance of nutrition and movement—that they're not applying in their daily lives.

We also have a lot of health experts and health professionals who may know (or think they know) a lot about health, but are they practicing what they preach?

Truth be told, to improve our health, we need to learn more about health in general. But we also need to apply what we've learned to our own lifestyle—to become self experts—because learning and applying are two very different things. If we want to see real results in our life, we must find harmony between the two.

This book is for modern-day, health-conscious consumers who want to see results in their lives. Maybe not by being "perfect" all the time, but by focusing on making progress and finding balance in their approach.

- What has been your health story in the past?
- What are your intentions for your health future?

The choice is yours.

Just as Morpheus offers Neo the choice between two futures in the form of the red pill and the blue pill in *The Matrix*, we have the opportunity to make decisions, with this book and inside each and every present moment, that will impact the future of our health and human experience.

Your current level of health, energy, happiness, and overall quality of life are by-products of the habits, environment, and overall lifestyle design you've lived in the past and are living in the present.

- Are you happy with those results?
- Are there opportunities to tweak the design of your lifestyle to bring about better, healthier habits?
- How are you called to evolve your own self-care and health care strategy so you can elevate your state?

We can all elevate our state of health and performance—if we just listen to our hearts and bodies, ask for help, and, sometimes, just get out of our own damn way.

Ok, my wrist is hurting. Time to move. Time to breathe.

Health from the heart, my friends. It's my art. And may it be yours as well.

Stay hungry. Stay blessed. And enjoy the quest.

Your friend and fellow health hacker,

TJ Anderson

Clinical Health Coach

Founder, Elevate Your State

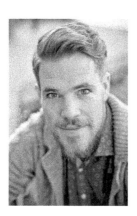

HOW TO USE THIS BOOK

Da Vinci, Our Stories, and the Artist in All of Us

All children are artists. The problem is how to remain an artist once he grows up.
— Pablo Picasso

Welcome da Vinci From Stage Left

Leonardo da Vinci serves as a model for what is possible when it comes to human achievement, and, perhaps more simply, being creative. His life story and his creations, such as the Vitruvian Man, can teach us a lot about approaching life's most important subjects. This includes our most important asset—our health.

Da Vinci was born to middle-class parents who were unmarried, and the stigma of "illegitimacy" stuck with him most of his life. He couldn't attend University, he couldn't pursue noble career paths, and he lacked formal education. Instead, he chose to study many things on his own, outside of a formal educational model. He initiated what would later be known as habitual autodidacticism, or learning about a subject independently, rather than through formal education.

He *chose* to learn. He *chose* to experiment. He *chose* to create. In addition to studying Latin and physics, da Vinci taught himself about human anatomy by dissecting cadavers so he could paint more true to the human form. He didn't just learn about a subject by reading about it, he learned by *doing*.

Here's the thing—we don't have control of the family or life situation into which we are born. The power of choice in childhood is limited compared with that of adulthood. But as we grow into teenagers, young adults, and eventually mature adults, we have the opportunity to start making more and more choices and to take personal responsibility for our lives—what we want to learn and what we want to achieve. We may not choose our life situations, but like da Vinci, we can certainly choose the life we want to create within each new moment.

Earn your diploma in Experimentation and your master's degree in Experience as you teach yourself about all the aspects of life that are most interesting to you.

The choices we have as consumers have never been as robust as they are today. At times, our options can be terribly overwhelming, especially when it comes to our health. As life throws us one obligation after another, both in our work and our families, how can we ensure we're taking care of ourselves and making healthy decisions? We were all raised in different families, with different ways of approaching our health. Perhaps you grew up with great, healthy habits as a kid. Or, like a lot of us, perhaps you didn't.

Either way, we have the choice *today* to experiment in an artful way to figure out how we can best improve our health as adults.

We don't lack the science, information, or technology to live healthy. We lack the art to know how to use them properly.

Our Health Today

It's no secret that, in general, our country's health is very poor. We've never been this fat or sick and now we're finally paying the price as a country. In 2014, *The Lancet*, one of the world's leading independent medical journals, published the results of a meta-analysis of 1,749 published studies on body weight from around the world. And the results may or may not surprise you. In the US, 70.9

percent of men and 61.9 percent of women were **overweight**, compared with 36.9 percent of men and 38 percent of women worldwide.

Another way to look at the alarming state of health in the US is to consider how much money we spend on health care compared with the rest of the world. In 2009, Oliver Uberti and the *National Geographic* released data comparing the average life expectancy in different countries with what each nation spends on health care per person. Life expectancy in the US was found to be seventy-eight years, which was comparable to that of the other countries; however, our health care spending per person was nearly double that of other advanced countries. Yes, double. Pretty startling to consider.

For what we're spending on health care, we don't seem to be getting a good return on our investment in terms of life expectancy.

So, what is the cause of poor health in the US? People sometimes blame it on a broken health care system or even a broken food system, and they aren't wrong. In fact, improving these two industries represents some of the greatest opportunities for positive change. The truth is, there isn't one right answer. But typically, poor health is related to lifestyle (i.e., habits and behaviors) and our environment.

Adults usually have some sort of general knowledge about the types of food, drink, and habits that are healthy. But in a world filled with so much information about the newest health foods, diet crazes, and "bio hacks," how can we keep up?

- How do we create clarity around where we are at currently in our health?
- How do we consider changing our behaviors and moving forward to establish healthier habits?

You see, like da Vinci, we have likely not followed a formal curriculum to learn what it takes to live healthy in today's society. Furthermore, some of the information we did learn as children or young adults may very well have been misinformation.

Let's face it: The world is changing right before our eyes. We are seeing technology change at an accelerated rate. The internet and emerging technologies are changing the way people answer questions and make decisions about their health. There is also more information available than ever before, simultaneously creating a culture of awareness and confusion. We are able to get things done a lot faster. And we often believe that makes our lives easier. But with this growth and speed mindset also comes the notion that we must always be working. Many of us are burning the candle at both ends, which restricts our ability to live with the health, peace, and performance we desire. Sometimes we miss the connection between our ability to live a healthy, balanced life and our ability to be successful in our work and in our relationships.

And if we are lucky enough to have the awareness to slow down, take a step back, and invest more in ourselves and our own health, how do we begin? And how do we sustain these changes?

- How do we find a balance between our health, our work, and our relationships?
- How do we handle our health effectively in this new, ever-changing era of technology?

There are now over fifty thousand health apps available to the average smartphone owner. But we have only one human body. One mind. One heart. And one relationship we must get right before our relationships with others can begin to flourish—the relationship with ourselves.

The Problem is the Opportunity

There is an opportunity that has gone almost unnoticed as a solution to fixing our country's epidemic of poor health and chronic, preventable disease.

And that's **personal health empowerment.**

You may be wondering, "What exactly do you mean by personal health empowerment, TJ?" I'm glad you asked.

This is my definition of personal health empowerment:

> *The process of communicating with ourselves and others in a way that helps us discover our own ideas and create a path of personal health optimization rooted in sustainable behavior change.*

In my health coaching experiences, I have found the concept of personal health empowerment to be crucial to client success. If the goal is to improve your health and become the best version of yourself through long-term, sustained, healthy behavior change, you must take the reins for your health.

Notice the focus is on *empowering* individuals, not telling them what to do. Telling people what to do is not what health coaching is about. That's not what behavior change is about. That's not what will help our country get out of this mess of sickness and disease. And that's not what I will do in this book. I'm not going to expect you to be perfect, either. I've actually learned that's the exact opposite goal or intention to carry, and it's not what long-term, sustainable success is all about.

You can pick up any health book on meditation, nutrition, movement, sleep, or relationships and it will tell you what you *should* be doing. It would reference the latest and greatest science to explain exactly why you should consider integrating that piece of information into your lifestyle. In fact, I will profile a few of those books within this book. But I won't tell you what you should do. I will share a framework and different lens through which you can consider approaching your life and your health journey. A lens of optimal health.

No matter where we are today as individuals, there is an opportunity to make a choice. We have an opportunity to choose ourselves and our own health and well-being to take our health to the next level.

Put simply, there is no blueprint for managing our own personal health. But I believe we can take a page out of da Vinci's book, and crack our own creative code to figure out what we can do to take control of our own health and performance.

Becoming a Health Hacker

When people ask me what it means to be a health hacker, I usually smile because it's a sign I've caught their attention and piqued their interest to learn or discover something new—a different way of looking at their health.

There are several key principles that distinguish those who are generally interested in learning about health from those who are ready to learn and experiment. That is, to become a health hacker, taking action when appropriate and learning from his or her experience.

- Developing the **Skill** of building your own holistic health care team
- Cultivating the **Willingness** to take action when appropriate and try new things
- Discovering the **Courage** to slow down the mind, get into the body and heart, and get real with how you feel
- Living with **Acceptance** of yourself and others, no matter how tempted you are to pass judgment in one way or another

Understanding and applying these principles can dramatically shift how we approach our life and our health, and in return, the quality of our life experience. We will explore all of these principles in the chapters that follow.

But until then, just know this—

I'm here to make the complex simple.

This book is my art from my heart and I appreciate you being here. It's taken some courage for me to share what I've learned and experienced. And I appreciate the courage it will take for you to explore your own health while reading about my journey as a self coach and a health coach. I respect your time and intend to provide you with a new perspective as you approach your health.

We Are Different—Together

No matter where you're at on the health spectrum and no matter your experiences in the health care system, you are welcome here.

Maybe you're a pro biohacker focused on optimizing your health. If so, welcome. In this book, you will find a solid review of ways to optimize your health and energy and maybe learn a few new "hacks" to add to your arsenal along the way.

Maybe you're not a pro biohacker, but are interested in taking your health, energy, and overall performance to the next level. Welcome. This book has your name written all over it.

You might be chomping at the bit to learn about some new tools or "health hacks" to add to your daily routine. Or maybe you're tired of trying to improve and want to take a break from trying to get better. Either way, welcome. I'm so glad you're here.

We may be at different points on the health and vitality spectrum, but we *all* have the potential to become health-conscious consumers, waking up to new areas of opportunity to make healthier decisions and treat our bodies, hearts, and minds with a little more TLC. As individuals, as communities, and as humans, we're called to evolve and explore new ways of being and living on the way to a higher quality experience.

To be clear, this is not a book about separation. While there are different levels of experience, knowledge, and states of health and well-being we all currently rest at as individuals, we don't have to feel or think we are separate from each other. This book is about connecting the ideas, relationships, and resources to support each other in understanding where we are in this moment of our lives and to ask some important questions:

- Where do we want to go?
- How can we use these connections to uplift ourselves and our human species, together?
- What else is possible in our health and performance?
- How can we prevent poor health and energy outcomes and stress less while still staying focused on our work, family, and relationships?

With a consistent thirst for growth, learning, and intentional self-experimentation…

I am convinced that you can learn to build
a lifestyle filled with less stress, more energy, and
VIBRANT health.

The Main Goal and Premise of this Book

Many people are influenced by marketing messages and new health trends that have them take action to improve their health. While this is not necessarily bad, it is important to consider whether these messages and health trends lay the proper foundation for human health. Do they help us create a sustainable approach to our health, integrating new behaviors and knowledge into our lifestyle—seamlessly and for the long term? Or do they only focus on short-term health kicks?

I don't just care about your ability to be successful with a short-term health goal or new health trend. Don't get me wrong—short-term health goals can be powerful and important for an overall health strategy. But like a beautiful Victorian mansion, unless you lay a strong foundation of fundamentals, your house of habits will crumble to the ground.

Let me be clear about one thing: Health hacking is a process. It's an art. But most of all, it's a journey, not a destination. The journey *is* the goal.

My goal is to empower true, sustainable health freedom for you, the health-conscious consumer. To look at your health through a new lens. And for the results to show.

Be Your Own Health Coach

When it comes to balancing and mastering the fundamental areas of our health and our ability to change and improve, this just might be one of the most important books you will read.

I know I'm biased, but I've spent the past seven years experimenting with what works and what doesn't, searching for the elusive happy-medium we call balance. I've been researching and applying the most important health practices I can find to create sustainable behavior change, both in my life and the lives of the clients I've served.

I'm writing this book from my experience in three areas:

- As a health coach, I have supported hundreds of people (entrepreneurs, business leaders, family, and friends) to establish sustainable, healthy habits and reach desired outcomes.

- As a team member of a health coach training organization, I have helped train thousands of health professionals to become behavior change specialists. As an ambassador for health in general, I have helped amplify the mission and message of some of the top brands in the health and biohacking space.
- And as a self coach and hacker of my own health, I have worked through my own issues and ego to heal suppressed emotions. I've built a best-in-class health care team to help fix key injuries and optimize my blood work. Perhaps most importantly, I've learned how to live a high-performance, yet low-stress lifestyle by listening to my body, establishing healthy habits, and trying new self-care strategies as needed.

So what does this mean for you?

Here's the deal. I'll walk you through what health hacking is about. If you want to be told what to do, find a consultant or a trainer. They would be happy to tell you what to do.

This book is about guiding you through specific questions that will help steer your thought process, create self-awareness, and establish sustainable behavior change so YOU can discover what works best for you to reach the health and performance you desire.

Together, we will define, learn about, and apply what we call optimal health. I'll help you understand your personal health blueprint, how to reset it, and how you can properly integrate changes into your health and lifestyle without negatively impacting your current lifestyle. In fact, these changes will do the exact opposite!

You'll learn from some of my favorite, go-to experts for optimizing health—Dave Asprey, JJ Virgin, and Ben Greenfield, to name a few.

And you'll learn some of the personal health hacks I use on a daily basis, not just to stay healthy, but to amplify mental performance in my work.

The Book Layout

Let's get creative and imagine our lives as a movie or a play. You are the main character, you are the director, and you are the writer. You are in charge of every major theme and detail of this piece. You are the artist who commands creative control.

What might your life-movie look like?

Every time I hear that question, it gets me thinking. I've always loved movies and plays, but I've never seen my life as one—until now. And what's great about this exercise is that it doesn't have to be perfect. I've got the ability to write, direct, and, perhaps more importantly, act out the film of the life that I choose to live. And so do you.

As with many movies and plays, this book is organized into different sections. Aristotle believed every piece of poetry or drama must have three parts—a beginning, middle, and end. Shakespeare preferred a five-act structure for his plays. In honor of the inspiring William Shakespeare, this book is organized in five acts:

- **Act 1–The Exposition: The setting is established, characters are developed, and conflict is introduced with a DRAMATIC question.**

   In Act 1, "Setting The Stage: The Future of Health is Already Here," we will begin by discussing our country's past and future health, highlighting key trends happening both inside and outside of the traditional health care system. We will also discuss how we're called to evolve our definition of health and get clear on our own story in our own lives. The goal isn't to simply *improve* ourselves all the time. Sometimes we need to *approve* of ourselves and where we're at in this moment.

- **Act 2–The Rising Action: This act will eventually lead you to the climax in Act 3. It is common for complications to arise in this act, or for the protagonist to experience obstacles that must be overcome.**

   In Act 2, "The Rise of the Optimized: Health Hackers Unite!", we will look closer at trends happening in the Biohacking and Quantified-Self movements. The obstacles that must be overcome? Managing the overwhelming amounts of science, information, and technology innovation while taking action in the most effective way possible to achieve personal health optimization. We'll get clear on what the Health Hacking approach actually entails and how it serves as an artful, simple solution to manage all areas of our health. This is when we start looking at some the latest and greatest behavior change science—and art, of course. Because where you find art, you will find action and, thus, results.

- **Act 3–The Climax: This is the turning point in a play, characterized by the highest amount of suspense.**

  In Act 3, "Behind the Scenes: The Inner Game of Health and Healing," we will start to get clear on the importance of getting better at *feeling* and not simply trying to *feel* better. What matter most are the stories we tell ourselves that hold us back from the people we're called to become. Everything changes after this act, because we realize it's not just about *doing*, but about the power of *being*; realizing who we are and who we want to become. I'll share some personal stories about body-image issues related to modeling, as well as ending up in the ER for low sodium. We will start to reflect on our lives and tap into our minds and hearts to do some major healing from childhood to today. The present moment is offered as a gateway to improved health, awareness, and peace of mind.

- **Act 4–The Falling Action: The story is coming to an end and any unknown details or plot twists are revealed and resolved.**

  In Act 4, "Getting Started: Take Inventory and Take Action," we will create a plan to initiate sustainable action in our health. We'll look at the most important areas of our health to measure (e.g., blood work, genetics, and behaviors) to create a plan for approaching our routines and habits, as well as setting goals on a daily, weekly, and monthly basis. The purpose? To prevent low energy, fatigue, and sickness, as well as to create more opportunities for flow states—when we both feel our best and perform our best, reaching new levels of joy in our lives. We'll end this act discussing the value of asking for help and ultimately building our own health care team, rooted in true and holistic health, wellness, and prevention.

- **Act 5–The Resolution: This is the outcome of the drama where the final message, moral, or lesson is shared.**

  In Act 5, "The Health Hacker Process and Game Plan," we'll explore some of my favorite health hacks, from health behaviors like sleep, movement, and nutrition, to state changers like cold showers, Wim Hof deep breathing, and float tanks. We'll also discuss top supplements, nootropics, and technologies I use to optimize my health. We'll make a plan for the health care team we've started to build, with a focus on maintaining a path of learning and growth for our health. Finally, we'll end with a major lesson to learn in our world today—have fun, disconnect from technology, and reconnect with nature.

This book is a blueprint for the modern day, health-conscious consumer. This is a call to action for each of us to become more personally responsible for ourselves, to support each other as we approach our health from a holistic point of view, and to understand that this life is truly a journey, not a destination.

In the words of da Vinci himself, "I have been impressed with the urgency of doing. Knowing is not enough; we must apply. Being willing is not enough; we must do."

Are you ready to explore new areas of yourself and reach your next level health?

If so, get ready for an adventure. You're in for a wild ride!

Before You Start Hacking

So what might you consider doing before you start reading this book?

1. Start to consider that this is not a short-term, quick-fix type of an approach. This is all about sustainability and finding joy in your approach. If you feel like you have a lot of opportunity to improve your

health, don't rush the change. Take action where you're called to, but don't overdo it. And if this sustainable approach to health optimization doesn't resonate with you, if just reading or listening to this section of the book creates tension for you and you want to stop reading, please know I welcome you. I honor you. And I invite you to stay for a while— or at least through the first two acts so you can get to the drama. You never know what you will learn.

2. Realize this isn't just about your health as you know and relate to it today. It's about something much different. We're talking about using your health as an asset in your overall life performance. So you don't just *look* good, but you *feel* and *function* on an entirely new level. We're talking true mental clarity, heightened focus when you want it, peace and calm when you want it, and an overall sense of well-being. Maybe you just want to live a long life in minimal pain and with better energy. Whatever your goal or interest is in life, your health can help you get there.

   • If you're a CEO, business owner, entrepreneur, or freelancer, how can your health and energy serve as an asset in your business?

   • If you're a part-time or full-time worker for another company, how can you optimize your health and performance to be more successful in your career, minimize your health risks, and just feel better?

   • If you're raising a family, how can you take care of yourself and your own health while also helping your kids become more health-conscious individuals in the process?

3. Third, pause for a moment and just breathe. Go ahead. Close your eyes. Take three deep breaths in this moment. And just feel whatever you're feeling.

Breathe.

Breathe.

Breathe.

As you breathe, feel and notice your breath, your body, and whatever else it is you feel and notice. Your breath is your secret weapon to building more conscious, intentional, present-moment awareness, and reaching the level of peace and performance you desire.

As we move forward in this book, **keep breathing**. It may sound simple, but conscious breathing deep into your lungs and your stomach will help you stay awake and alert. The result? You'll be more attentive and prepared to integrate what you're learning about yourself and your health into your life. Let's make the most of it—together.

May we give thanks for our breath and the overall health we have right now. It's only going to get better.

Welcome, my friends. It's great to have you here.

Now let's get hacking!

Your Friends are Waiting

Join the Private Group on Facebook to Book Club this book! Just search for **"The Health Hacker Book Club"** on Facebook and request access. Your request will be approved and you can start connecting with your friends and fellow health hackers about the book! Plus, if you'd like to unlock exclusive access to tools and resources to support you throughout this book, go to www.healthhackerbook. com/bookclub.

ACT 1

Setting The Stage:

The Future of Health is Already Here

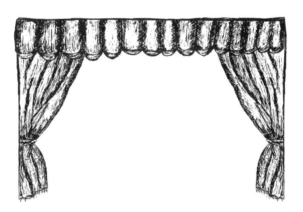

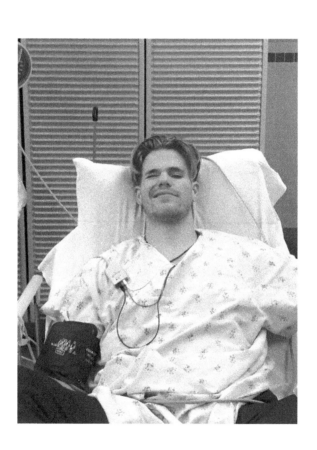

CHAPTER 1

Goodbye, Sick-Care; Hello, Self-Care:

Your Health is in Your Hands

*You never change things by fighting the existing reality.
To change something, build a new model that makes
the existing model obsolete.*
– BUCKMINSTER FULLER

The first time I visited the ER, I was about three years old and had just overdosed on an entire bottle of Children's Tylenol. Yes, an entire bottle. Was it my fault? Nope. My babysitter reportedly told me it was candy in order to get me to take it for a high fever. But did I learn from it? Heck no! I was three, for goodness' sake, and was duped into an accidental poisoning!

The last time I visited the ER was in February 2015 for what health experts call hyponatremia (low sodium and electrolytes) after passing out at brunch with my family. At twenty-seven years old, I was a full-grown adult who was already pretty experienced and knowledgeable about my health. In fact, I was a year and a half into writing the book you have in your hands right now and about ready to hit "SEND" to my editor. You see, I thought the book I'd been writing for the past few years was about finished. But sometimes God, the Universe, and life in general takes you down a path that you don't plan; forces you to wake up and shows you what you need most. At least that's what I realized after surviving this near-death experience.

The details of my visit to the ER—like how it happened and how it spurred nearly two more years of writing this book—will be revealed later. But until then, know this: My ER experience was my ultimate wake-up call in life to this point, through which I finally realized how my health and my entire life was really in my own hands. I could receive reactive help from the health care system, but if I wanted to truly optimize my health and live a healthy and happy life for the long haul, I would need to say "goodbye" to sick-care and "hello" to self-care. I could take ultimate responsibility for my own health and inspire others in the process.

Because our health really is in our own hands.

Sick-Care System

When you think about our health care system, what comes to mind? Perhaps you've been treated in hospitals or clinics. Or perhaps you've experienced many different health care settings with your family or friends as patients.

Either way, I'm willing to bet the majority of memories from your health care system experience are not completely happy and positive. Often times, they're quite sad and emotional. But the health care system isn't broken, it's changing. There are new movements starting to reverse the previous model of health care. Movements where patients are in the drivers' seat, feeling empowered and confident in their health, and the care team is more focused on proactive self-care, as opposed to reactive sick-care.

While working in and around personal health coaching, group fitness training, community and corporate wellness, and population health management for hospitals and medical groups, I've seen a lot. Modern medicine and advanced technologies in the United States can do amazing things, but often our health care system has very little to do with health. A majority of people don't access the formal health care system as we know it to *stay* healthy. As my mentor and Executive Director of the Iowa Chronic Care Consortium, Dr. Bill Appelgate, often says, "Much of health care is organized and delivered to mend the broken, treat the ill, and cure the sick. Not to help us stay healthy."

In fact, if we're honest with ourselves, it isn't a health care system that works to develop health. It's a sick-care system and it always has been.

But this isn't a book about a giant health care system or sick-care system. This is a book about showcasing the latest innovations in health care and self-care, and what that means for you as a modern-day, health-conscious consumer.

Throughout this book you'll learn a lot about how organizations like the Iowa Chronic Care Consortium are leading the way in innovating our health care system. But until then, know this:

Self-care isn't just the future of health care. It's already here. And it can be your greatest asset—if you let it.

In order for you to understand why innovation in health care is relevant to you, we must dive a bit deeper. Let's set the stage by looking at how our health care system started and what that means for us today.

What is "Health Care" and How did it Start?

Health care is defined by Merriam-Webster Dictionary as "efforts made to maintain or restore physical, mental, or emotional well-being especially by trained licensed professionals." But how did it start?

The United States health care system started out of need. When individuals had a episodic or acute illnesses that drove them to a place of very poor health, they needed help. And as more and more hospitals were created and more and more doctors learned about the science of the human body, opportunities to receive help grew. Most doctors and other health professionals were taught and trained to treat disease and poor health outcomes through the use of medications and procedures in an attempt to mend the broken and cure the sick.

Whereas acute illnesses (e.g., pneumonia, influenza, and tuberculosis) are episodic and short-term, chronic health conditions (e.g., heart disease, chronic obstructive pulmonary disease (COPD), and diabetes) usually don't go away. You can have diabetes for multiple years of your life, but you're likely not going to have the flu for multiple years. You get the idea.

Note: You don't have to have one of these chronic diseases to experience chronic conditions in your life. For example, you may have chronic stress, chronic fatigue, or chronic pain. These aren't diseases, necessarily, but they still have an impact on health and are largely preventable. More on that later.

Herein lies a looming problem within our country's health care system. While the US health care system was designed to primarily address acute illness, **our country's biggest health care problem is no longer acute illness. It's chronic disease.** But our health care system wasn't really built for chronic disease, and historically, many health care professionals were not trained to promote health.

Perhaps what's worse, our current health care system and some health care providers don't begin to scratch the surface of promoting behaviors one might embrace to prevent illness or improve and maintain health.

What Causes Chronic Disease?

There are several reasons why our country (and our entire world) has seen a dramatic spike in poor health and, specifically, chronic disease. We could talk about our broken food system, changes to our environment, our government getting the nutrition guidelines wrong (for, well, the past 40 years), or rapid technology innovation that is creating a culture of convenience mixed with an addiction to technologies like television, smartphones, and social media.

I could talk for hours on this issue and we'll definitely cover it more throughout this book. But at the end of the day, our level of health and the cause of chronic disease can be traced back to one thing—our behaviors. In fact, some people tend to use the term "lifestyle disease" instead of chronic disease to showcase how disease is linked to the style of life you live.

The System is Not Broken, It's Outdated

A lot of people say our health care system is broken; however, when we say something is broken, we usually mean it was once working and is no longer working at the same capacity. That it was created properly in the first place. In my opinion, the quote, "Every system is perfectly designed to get the results it gets" is worth considering. Our health care system is not broken, my friends. It's simply an outdated, inefficient model.

Western medicine is necessary to address acute, unplanned health issues. But it is not always the best route to follow if we want prevent disease and optimize health. This is how other top health and fitness leaders see the topic as well. I had a chance to interview Ben Greenfield, founder of top health blog and podcast at https://BenGreenfieldFitness.com about how he views western medicine:

> The emergency room is a good place to go if you break your arm or if your head gets run over by a car. But if you have some sort of general wellness or lifestyle issue such as a gut pathology, I'd encourage you to see a Chinese herbal medicinal formulator or a functional medicine practitioner or a good naturopathic doctor instead of, say, lounging around in a hospital, taking pharmaceuticals, or using western medicine based antibiotics.

The traditional US health care system may not always be the best solution to every health concern, and it isn't the most efficient system either. It's often said that a third of US health care spending is wasted. According to a 2010 report from the Institute of Medicine (IOM), an estimated $750 billion to $765 billion was wasted on unnecessary health care services in 2009. Pure waste.

The traditional health care system is bankrupting our country. We need to end the old model of reacting to disease in our current sick-care system, and embrace a new model of true prevention and even prediction. We can't rely on a system acting like a catcher's mitt for disease anymore. It's time to evolve our health care system.

Welcome to Precision Medicine

While there are a lot of activities we, as consumers, can do on our own to support the evolution of health care, it's also helpful to know what our government and top scientific organizations are doing to support that end. In January 2015, President Obama announced a new focus for health care with the Precision Medicine Initiative:

Through collaborative public and private efforts, the Precision Medicine Initiative will leverage advances in genomics, emerging methods for managing and analyzing large data sets while protecting privacy, and health information technology to accelerate biomedical discoveries. The Initiative will also engage a million or more Americans to volunteer to contribute their health data to improve health outcomes, fuel the development of new treatments, and catalyze a new era of data-based and more precise medical treatment.

This announcement is only the beginning of health care innovation. In his book, *The Patient Will See You Now,* Dr. Eric Topol discusses how people can take unlimited blood pressures or blood glucose measurements, or even do an electrocardiogram (EKG or ECG) via their smartphone.

The first time I had an ECG emailed to me by a patient, with the subject line, "I'm in atrial fib, now what do I do?", I immediately knew that the world had changed. The patient's phone hadn't just recorded the data—it had interpreted it!

This is a real example of innovation at its best. To showcase another example, let's take a look at one of the most cutting-edge organizations in the country to see innovation in action.

Sequencing the human genome was no easy task. When Craig Venter, co-founder and executive chairman of Human Longevity Inc. (HLI), and his team first sequenced the human genome in 2000, it cost an estimated $100 million. But today it's possible to sequence the human genome for $1,000. According to Venter,

If we can predict and know at birth—or even before birth—our risk of cancer, heart disease, dementia, or different genetic diseases, at a stage where you might be able to do something about them even before they occur, that's going to be a whole paradigm shift in medicine.

This development speaks to how quickly we're innovating in this country, creating a wave of precision medicine that's only growing. What's really possible with precision medicine?

Well, Peter Diamandis, co-founder of HLI, believes a lot.

Based out of San Diego, California, HLI's first health center, The Health Nucleus, is a data-hub focused on extending the healthy human lifespan. In fact, it's one of the largest health data mining projects in human history. Cutting-edge technology is being used to digitize the human body through the collection of DNA sequence data, microbiome and metabolomics, as well as full body and brain scans.

The goal? To understand the correlation between people's genomics and health outcomes. Or according to Diamandis, the goal is to **"make healthcare predictive and preventative."**

The other side of their business—the stem cell side—is focused on learning how to rejuvenate stem cells. This is where the possibilities get interesting, and the science complex. Here's an excerpt of what Diamandis shared on a recent episode of *The Tim Ferriss Show*:

> As we get older, our stem cell population does two things. One, it begins to dwindle and our stem cell reserves get reduced. The second is our stem cells undergo these epigenetic changes, these mutations, deletions, insertions. And our stem cells become less and less able to repair our body's injured tissues. So, one of the ideas for Human Longevity Inc. is can we in fact extract your stem cells, identify what epigenetic changes have taken place, repair your stem cells, proliferate them, provide them back to you, and restore your regenerative engine. **So our mission is to extend the healthy human lifespan thirty or forty years. To make one-hundred years old the new sixty.**

HLI is ahead of the curve. It is driving a shift in health care innovation and creating a new model for precision medicine, monitoring health and treating disease before it occurs. And it's here to stay.

Believe the Behaviors: The 80–80–80 Rule

Earlier in my career, I spent two years working as a consultant for a health care non-profit organization called the Iowa Chronic Care Consortium (ICCC). Based out of Des Moines, Iowa, ICCC has done large-scale, population health work for more than a decade. This organization is 100 percent committed to changing behaviors one patient at a time through *The Clinical Health Coach Training*, a best-in-class health coach training developed for front-line health professionals. For two years, I learned the ins and outs of health coaching in health care, working with large health systems and medical groups across the country to deploy this health coach training.

The goal? To equip front-line health professionals, such as physicians, social workers, nurses and care coordinators, with the health coaching communication skills they need to become behavior change specialists with their patients.

Dr. Bill Appelgate, founder of the Clinical Health Coach explains:

> The power of health coaching is to do three things: (1) Improve health behaviors, (2) build self-care skills, and (3) inspire ongoing accountability on the part of the patient. We must see the patient as capable. At the end of the day that's our game-changing strategy if we want to make big improvements in health care.

In this health coach training, there is a popular way of explaining the prevention and management of chronic conditions called the 80–80–80 Rule.

- 80 percent or more of health care dollars are spent on chronic illness
- 80 percent or more are spent on high cost (and often preventable) services (e.g., hospitalizations, readmissions, ED visits)
- 80 percent or more of health care is self-care

These statistics are a bit startling. But they are necessary to understand when we look at creating a new model to improving health care.

Salutogenesis—The Need for a New Approach

As discussed earlier, our traditional health care system in the US is mostly a sick-care system, where professionals are trained to understand and focus on the origin and development of disease. This particular model of training is called pathogenesis. Pathogenesis still plays a critical role in treating people who are working through acute and episodic illness. If it weren't for pathogenesis, we wouldn't have the medical breakthroughs and treatments we have today.

However, most pathogenic approaches don't address the true, root causes of disease.

As a result, a majority of our health care professionals don't always have the time, training, or resources to explore all of the factors that play a role in one's disease process.

And when we combine these issues with a fundamentally flawed fiscal model in our health care system—incentivizing the treatment of symptoms with a "quick fix" pill or injection—we have a recipe for disaster, at least in our health.

While working with Dr. Appelgate, I learned about a new model of training to compliment our pathogenic model within health care—salutogenesis. Salutogenesis is a term coined by Aaron Antonovsky, a professor of medical sociology. In his book, *Health, Stress and Coping*, Antonovsky posits that life experiences help shape one's sense of coherence; life is understood as more or less comprehensible, meaningful, and manageable. A strong sense of coherence helps one utilize their resources to cope with stressors and tension successfully.

The word salutogenesis comes from "salus," meaning health in Latin, and "genesis," meaning the origin of something. Therefore, salutogenesis is based on the origin and creation of health.

So, instead of looking at how or why disease happened and treating it accordingly (pathogenesis), salutogenesis provides us with an empowering model to understand the factors that support and create human health and well-being in the first place.

In my opinion, an optimal approach to health restoration in our society would involve the right balance of a properly functioning pathogenic model (understanding and responding to the *true root causes* of dis-ease) and a salutogenic model (understanding the origin and creation of holistic health-ease).

At the end of the day, if we as consumers desire a model where we are sick as little as possible, we might want to focus on what leads to health in the first place. And that starts at the most fundamental level with self-care.

So what is self-care, exactly? And how do we impact health care spending and preventable health conditions through behavior change in our own lives?

The Self-Care Solution: The What and the Why

There are many definitions of self-care, but the World Health Organization's definition is especially good:

> **Self-care is what people do for themselves to establish and maintain health, and to prevent and deal with illness.** It is a broad concept encompassing hygiene (general and personal), nutrition (type and quality of food eaten), lifestyle (sporting activities, leisure), environmental factors (living conditions, social habits) socio-economic factors (income level, cultural beliefs), and self-medication.

Even if you aren't experiencing chronic disease right now, the concept of self-care is still very important. The truth is, we all deal with self-care on some level, in our lives or in the lives of our family members. The choices we make related to our health all fall under the umbrella of self-care. And it's up to us to find the right balance between taking care of ourselves, our family, and our work.

But, with health care innovation happening so quickly, how do we keep up?

Should we wait (or even fight) for these changes to unfold within a poorly performing, reactive model of health care? Or could we build our own?

How do we build a self-coach approach with us in the driver's seat of our own health?

For starters, we must say "goodbye" to sick-care and "hello" to self-care. We can no longer be dependent on our current health care system and our medical doctors to keep us healthy. As the title of this book and this first chapter suggests, if we want to elevate our state of health and performance, we must claim responsibility and take our health in our own hands.

The stage is set. The characters are ready. Now it's time to act.

Summary:

- Our traditional health care system is essentially a sick-care system, focusing on the origin and treatment of dis-ease not the creation of health-ease.
- Many health care professionals who practice western medicine don't have the time, training, or resources to explore all of the factors that play a role in one's disease process.
- An optimal approach to health restoration in our society would involve the right balance between a properly functioning pathogenic model (understanding and responding to the true root causes of dis-ease) and a salutogenic model (understanding and responding to the creation of health-ease).
- Self-care is what people do for themselves to establish and maintain health, and to prevent and deal with illness.
- Health care isn't broken, it's changing. There are new models of health care focused on empowering patients to change their behaviors and actually treating the cause of illness and disease, not just the symptoms.
- With the smartphone, the future of health care is in your hands— literally.
- Organizations like Human Longevity Inc. are changing what's possible with disease prevention, precision medicine, and consumer-driven health care.

Action Items:

1. What does self-care mean to you?
2. How do you manage your health when you get sick or stressed out? Do you turn to your doctor, Google, or both? Do you take action on your own? Are there specific websites or blogs you like to use? Write out all the resources you use—from people and organizations to information and technology—to manage your health.
3. What type of health care professionals do you have in your life? Do they support you in understanding exactly what's going on in your body? Do they seem to simply treat your symptoms without addressing the cause?

We will discuss options in greater detail later in the book, but until then, take an inventory of who makes up your care team.

4. **BONUS**: Read *Where Does It Hurt? An Entrepreneur's Guide to Fixing Health Care* by Jonathan Bush, or *The Patient Will See You Now* by Dr. Eric Topol. These books will provide a deeper understanding of the history of the US health care system and, perhaps more importantly, the changes starting to unfold.

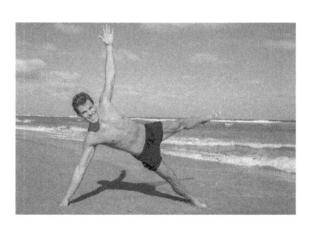

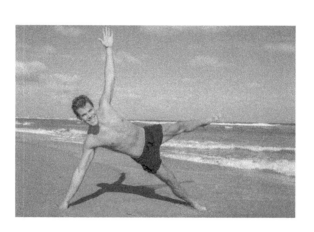

CHAPTER 2

Beyond The Physical:
Health Redefined

*We can't solve problems by using the same kind of thinking
we used when we created them.*
— ALBERT EINSTEIN

Since you're reading this book, it's probably safe to say you care about your health. And for good reason—your health is important. Without it, you are not able to fully experience the events, moments, and people you love most.

As health-conscious consumers, we understand our health is important. But what does it really mean to us? It seems like everyone has a slightly different definition of the word *health*. We create a story in our heads about what our health means to us based on our past experiences, and since we all come from different backgrounds and families, a multitude of definitions of health exist.

In this chapter, we will discuss some of the current, well-known definitions of health, we'll explore how we're called to evolve our health beyond the physical, and I'll share a fundamental framework to follow when asking the all-important question: **"How are we called to evolve our approach to health?"**

How are we called to evolve our approach to health?

When I first started down my personal path to improving my health, all I could think about was improving my fitness. I had the general knowledge and training that proper amounts of exercise and eating fewer processed foods and less sugar was good for me, but that's as far as my knowledge went. Perhaps I had some idea that getting restful sleep was important, but it wasn't a big focus in my health goals. Without even realizing it, the general concept of eating healthy and working out became my definition of health. My focus was solely on the external. I wanted to look better, so I started to "eat healthier" and get more workouts in, focusing 100 percent on the physical body. I was missing out on so much more.

Focusing on just the physical body to *look* good can be a great starting point, because we all start somewhere. But in my experience, it's not sustainable. I didn't think about how the other areas of my life were affecting my overall health—emotionally, mentally, and spiritually. My target was off and my approach was narrow-minded. The result? I didn't see the results I wanted. I didn't *feel* better, in fact I suffered a lot through the lens of my own judgment—constantly not feeling fit enough.

While being physically fit is very important, it is just one piece to the overall puzzle I was aiming to solve; I just didn't know it yet. In fact, it took me about three years in fitness and four months of modeling in Miami for this blind spot to reveal itself.

Health vs. Fitness Vanity: My Miami Modeling Adventures

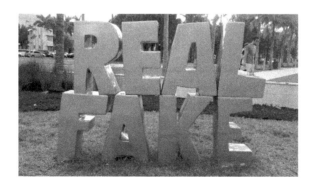

Here's the story of me meeting a photographer in Iowa and moving to Miami, Florida, to be a model.

After working and training in the health coaching and group fitness space, I met a photographer at church who was interested in learning more about my work. Over coffee, I learned she had some connections in the modeling industry and she thought I "had a look"—if I was interested, that is. After reflecting on it for a few weeks, I decided to take her up on her offer to introduce me to some of her colleagues. Before long, I joined one of the local modeling agencies in Des Moines, Iowa. This particular agency's business model was focused on finding and developing local, "raw" talent that could be placed in larger markets across the world. So, after six months of "working" on my body and getting in better shape, we submitted my photos to a few agencies. Before I knew it, an agency selected me and I was on a one-way flight to Miami.

I spent the first four months of 2014 as a model in sunny South Beach. As a health coach and fitness trainer from Iowa, I thought modeling would be an easy opportunity to make some side money and something that could be used as a platform to spread health and wellness to the world. But this twenty-five-year-old dude from Iowa was in for a culture shock.

The truth is, the modeling industry is not an easy place to work. I had an inspirational, feel-good reason for getting into modeling, but it didn't go as smoothly as I had planned. The money and work wasn't there. I experienced some financial stress. And I got caught up in the party scene, having a lot of fun drinking and dancing and flirting with beautiful women.

I started to feel like I was developing an online reputation that the average person couldn't relate to—that *I* couldn't relate to. The pictures and videos of beach parties made it seem like I was on spring break—a spring break that started in winter and lasted a couple of extra months. Miami, the modeling industry, and my experiences began to feel "real fake."

My values were starting to slip. I partied too hard and my body paid for it. I was in a vicious cycle of trying to achieve the perfect body while also partying my ass off. Here I thought I wouldn't get caught up in the glamour or perfection mindset of modeling, or all of the egos swimming through the streets of South Beach. But I was wrong.

There were also some memories I don't like to relive that really shook me up.

(CAUTION: The following content is real and raw. But hey, life happens. Thank you in advance for reserving your judgments and for your love and acceptance.)

One night, in particular, I decided to go out and network with someone important in the modeling industry. You see, I didn't have the best ten-pack body, so I was looking for any leg-up I could find. During this night of drinking and schmoozing, I let my guard and my values down. Before I knew it, I was given some white powder in the bathroom of a club. (And no, this wasn't grass-fed collagen protein or magnesium, my friends.) After this experience, I seriously don't remember much from the night. I just remember waking up in someone's apartment with a person who was influential in the modeling industry making a move on me. I was extremely uncomfortable and didn't know what to do. Except leave.

Was I raped? No.

Did I get drugged and black out in my ego's quest for triumph? Perhaps.

You might be wondering why I am sharing such a dark, scary, unfortunate story. The truth is, I share this story so other people can learn from it. This isn't the easiest story to share. But it's my truth. I need to get it off my chest. The modeling industry is not all sunshine and rainbows. I made poor choices, and was taken advantage of.

Thankfully, I learned valuable life lessons from this experience, which could have had a much worse ending. I'm grateful to be able to reflect on this. No matter our environment, it's easy to get caught up with the need to impress the people around us.

All in all, Miami was one hell of a ride for me, and I wouldn't change the overall experience for the world. Thankfully, after a few years of falling, growing, and learning about my ego, I've consciously created a new definition of and approach to health. One that is more heart-centered and holistic, integrating the mental, emotional, and spiritual elements of my life. But before we explore any more of my journey, let's take a look at how the word *health* came to be.

The Etymology of the Word *Health*

Understanding where words come from intrigues me. When we look at the word *health*, is it possible we don't always look at the whole picture of what health really means?

The word's origins are imbedded in a root word that also means whole and holy. According to naturopath Dr. Herbert Shelton, "When the English language as we know it today was borne in the 1300s, the Old English word root 'hal' evolved into three words: 'health,' 'whole,' and 'holy.' And at one time there was just the one word…'hal' to express these three concepts." Dr. Shelton goes on to explain the original meanings of these words:

> "Healing" is derived from the same root and means… "to restore to a state of wholeness, soundness, or integrity." "Holy" comes from the same root and signifies… "wholeness" and "purity of mind and spirit." Taken in its fullness of meaning, therefore, "health" has come to mean… "completeness and perfection of organization, fitness of life, freedom of action, harmony of functions, vigor and freedom from all stain and unholy corruption." The etymology of the word "health" is thus fascinating! In a phrase, "health" is… "A SOUND MIND AND SPIRIT IN A SOUND BODY!

> *To be Healthy…*
> *Is to be Whole…*
> *Is to be Holy…*

Making the connection between spirituality and health presents a powerful model for us to consider. Additionally, it is useful to explore how society defines health today.

Health Redefined

The word *health* often means something different to everyone who uses it. In my research, the most frequently quoted definition of health is from the World Health Organization (WHO) over half a century ago. According to the WHO, health is "a complete state of physical, mental and social well-being, and not merely the absence of disease or infirmity."

The WHO did a great job of putting this together. This definition of health gives credit to physical health, while also touching on mental health and social well-being. Furthermore, it goes on to say that health is "not merely the absence of disease." I love this, because it explicitly states that just because you don't have a disease, doesn't mean you are truly healthy. Our country has millions of people who don't have a sickness or disease, but are still be on their way to developing those outcomes.

After exploring improved health in my life and the lives of others, I've come up with a new way of looking at our health. Let's take a step back to see the bigger picture of what actually causes disease and poor health in the first place.

What factors play a role in one's symptoms or current state of health?

The Living Proof Institute, a functional medicine organization, created an illustration (as shown in figure 1) that depicts the role of root causes and dysfunctions in the development of poor health outcomes.

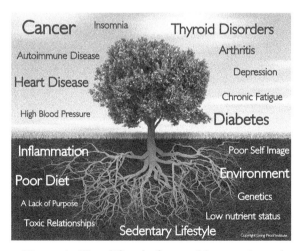

Figure 1. How lifestyle factors (the roots) produce health outcomes (the fruit).
Source: Reproduced by permission from The Living Proof Institute.

As you can see, the underlying issues placed in the roots of the tree are some root causes of disease. Not surprisingly, inflammation is known as one of the major causes of disease; however, something *causes* inflammation. It doesn't just happen on its own. **As highlighted by this Functional Tree, a true pathogenic model aims to address the origin (or causes) of disease, and not just the symptoms and corresponding treatment.**

To properly heal an organism as self-regulating as the human body, we must consider all the possible causes within a pathogenic model.

The Possibilities are Endless

When I first began intentionally learning about my health, I went through a health education curriculum called *Healthy for Life University*. The course materials included information about a well-known physician and pioneer in the field of epigenetics and genetic expression, Dr. Bruce Lipton. In his book, *The Biology of Belief*, Lipton discusses the recent science of how changes in genetic expression, rather than genetic code itself, relates to disease.

> Also featured in the book *Embrace, Release, Heal: An Empowering Guide to Talking About, Thinking About, and Treating Cancer* by Leigh Forston, Lipton says, "Our health is not controlled by genetics." Essentially, just because you have a gene for cancer, doesn't mean it has to be turned on. Researchers, including Lipton, have found that lifestyle and environment play key roles in our overall health, and both factors influence our genes. For example, data suggest 90 to 95 percent of cancer can be attributed to lifestyle and environment, or in other words, is 100 percent preventable.

Furthermore, and consistent with the idea in neuroscience that the subconscious mind controls 95 percent of our lives, Lipton believes that changing the way we *think* can actually influence our health outcomes:

> The function of the mind is to create coherence between our beliefs and the reality we experience. What that means is that your mind will

adjust the body's biology and behavior to fit with your beliefs. If you've been told you'll die in six months and your mind believes it, you most likely will die in six months. That's called the nocebo effect, the result of a negative thought, which is the opposite of the placebo effect, where healing is mediated by a positive thought.

Now, these statements may shock you. Or maybe it elicits some other emotion, as we've all lost family members to some sort of sickness or disease.

No matter what you believe or know about what's possible in your health, the emerging field of epigenetics is changing how we approach health with respect to prevention. It is starting to show both the medical community and consumers how much is possible in our health.

What does that mean for us as health hackers?

It means our genes don't run the game, but are only some of the players. It highlights how much is possible in creating the health we desire.

Now, you may be someone who currently has a sickness, disease, or other health condition, or maybe you've had one in the past. Either way, this realization presents an opportunity for us to tweak our approach to handling a sickness when it comes and also preventing it in the first place through healthy behaviors.

The Key to Health is Integration—Four Areas of Macro Health

Our total human experience evolves in an integrated manner. The head and the heart are always responding to the physical body, and the physical body is always responding to the experience of the head and the heart. And when we're dealing with illness or decisions that impact our health, we must deal with the body, mind, and heart in an integrated manner.

In my experience, the key to making healthy decisions involves integrating **Four Areas of Macro Health**:

1. Physical–Creating a strong and healthy body for greater vitality
2. Mental–Understanding our cognitive processes and how our brain works to be more present, focused, and optimistic

3. Emotional–Building emotional awareness and more positive relationships
4. Spiritual–Understanding your purpose in life and connecting in relationship with the divine; something greater than oneself

Note: If you are not a very spiritual person, that is OK. In fact, this book is not heavily focused on spirituality. While I talk about the impact God has made in my life and how we all may relate to spirituality, the focus is on how we can create a healthy journey in the physical world.

Ten Areas of Micro Health

Now that we've highlighted the Four Areas of Macro Health, let's take a look at the micro components influencing our current level of health:

1. Nutrition
2. Movement
3. Sleep
4. Relationships
5. Spirituality
6. Nature
7. Technology
8. Career and Purpose
9. Stress Management
10. Your Health Care

Integrative Health

Integrative Health is a state of being that involves the integration of body (physical), mind (mental), heart (emotional), and soul (spiritual).

If our goal is to be completely healthy and whole beings, we must begin by integrating these Four Areas of Macro Health and Ten Areas of Micro Health. We can focus on the physical all we want, but if we do not take into account the mental, emotional, and spiritual sides of our human experience, we will miss out on true health and wholeness.

Summary:

- The societal definition of health typically focuses on diet and fitness (physical health), and often ignores the mental, emotional, and spiritual elements of health.
- The key to overall health is the integration of our physical, mental, emotional, and spiritual health.
- Health is both a current state of being and the process or journey that leads to our health in the future.

Action Items:

How are you doing? As human beings, we have a great need to know we are making progress. It's how we're wired. Let's take an inventory of our Macro and Micro Health, remembering wherever you are right now is OK. We're all at a different levels of health, and the goal of this exercise is not to be critical of ourselves or to compare ourselves to others. The idea is to simply take inventory of our state of health and well-being right now, considering what's possible with some basic questions:

1. How often do you feel stressed, sad, or overwhelmed? How often are you sick, hungover (from food or alcohol), or in physical pain? How do these feelings and symptoms relate to your habits?
2. Do your food, drink, and supplement choices impact how you feel and perform?
3. Next, rate your level of health from 1 to 5 for each of the Four Areas of Macro Health and Ten Areas of Micro Health, where 1 is "poor" and 5 is "great." Then give yourself an overall Holistic Health Score, which shows a snapshot of your level of health based on both macro and micro areas of health.

   Note: We're not looking for an average of these four scores, but rather a general idea of how you think these areas of your life are operating—individually and together. For example, how does your mind respond to your feelings and emotions, and how do your emotions play a role in your physical health?

Here we go.

Macro Health

Physical	1 - 2 - 3 - 4 - 5
Mental	1 - 2 - 3 - 4 - 5
Emotional	1 - 2 - 3 - 4 - 5
Spiritual	1 - 2 - 3 - 4 - 5

Micro Health

Nutrition	1 - 2 - 3 - 4 - 5
Movement	1 - 2 - 3 - 4 - 5
Sleep	1 - 2 - 3 - 4 - 5
Relationships	1 - 2 - 3 - 4 - 5
Spirituality	1 - 2 - 3 - 4 - 5
Nature	1 - 2 - 3 - 4 - 5
Technology	1 - 2 - 3 - 4 - 5
Career & Purpose	1 - 2 - 3 - 4 - 5
Stress Management	1 - 2 - 3 - 4 - 5
Your Health Care	1 - 2 - 3 - 4 - 5

Holistic Health Score

Total	1 - 2 - 3 - 4 - 5

Throughout this book, we will explore these areas of health further, and will work to apply them to our daily habits. Until then, I hope this brief overview was helpful for you to check in with your bigger picture of health.

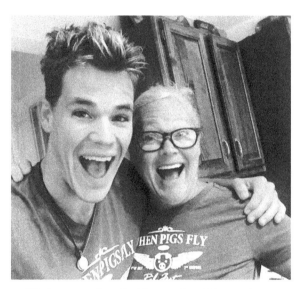

With my mother, Debbie, in Des Moines, Iowa.

CHAPTER 3

What's Your Story?

Approve Thy Self Before You Improve Thy Health

*Educating the mind without educating the heart
is no education at all.*

— ARISTOTLE

Kansas City, Missouri. 11:00 p.m., Friday, spring 2014

I was nervous and excited at the same time. I knew maybe seven of the twenty or more people at this so-called "heart-opening ceremony" and I didn't know what to expect.

I thought to myself, "Is this going to be an orgy? Is it going to turn into some sort of spiritual sex séance?" Nope. It was better than that.

The music played, the incense and candles burned, and one simple, yet profound conversation began to unfold.

As I sat across from a young woman whom I had never met, I mustered up the courage to share a very vulnerable part of myself.

I had just returned to the Midwest after modeling for four months in Miami. And so I decided to share how I struggled with feeling judged for my looks. I shared how I struggled with a perfection mindset as a model, whose 10 percent body fat and six-pack abs weren't good enough for the cameras.

This was what I had been through. This was how I felt.

She felt my pain. She felt my sadness. And she felt called to place six very powerful words on my heart that I will never forget; without them, I may not have written this book.

"You are more than your looks," she said. And she repeated, "You are more than your looks. You are more than your looks."

Those six words changed everything. I felt something I had never felt before.

My heart opened up and I felt free. I felt appreciated beyond my looks. I felt seen and accepted for who I was. I felt understood.

For someone who struggled with placing so much of my self-worth on how I looked (in the mirror or on camera), her six words were more important to me than any six-pack I could ever wish for. Her words, her eye contact, and her heart touched my heart. She shifted my energy from focusing on the physical to focusing on my heart.

Her acknowledgment meant the world to me. It allowed me to receive so much love, both from her and from myself. It unlocked something profound in my heart.

This heart-opening ceremony would mark the start of a twelve-month journey of self-love, self-acceptance, and self-approval.

Healing and Acceptance

In our world today, it's very easy to get caught up in the self-improvement movement. Have you been there? Where you want to work on or do better in an area of your health, work, or relationships, and all you can think is, "Am I good enough?"

This is one of the recurring questions that came up for me while modeling in Miami. Even looking in the mirror, I couldn't help but place judgment on myself and how I looked. In an industry where the focus is completely on appearance, feelings can easily take a backburner. It's funny, I just wanted to be seen for who I was—a healthy, fun-loving human being. But that's not what I experienced.

We all have our own stories. But here's the thing. There are actually multiple ways to look at the stories in our life. For example, my story of not being good enough in modeling was rooted in comparison, self-judgment, and the need to constantly "improve" myself.

I based so much of my identity on physical characteristics and so much of my energy on *improving* my physical body (as well as my financial bottom-line), that I lost sight of the value of *approving* of myself and loving myself unconditionally.

If you think about it, society does not always provide a path for developing a life rooted in unconditional love and acceptance. Often love and acceptance are taught through family. But as adults, we must *choose* the level of love and acceptance we want in our lives.

The heart-opening ceremony I attended is an example of how I chose to create unconditional love and self-acceptance in my life. But it doesn't end there. This was the start of my healing journey. Sometimes I feel like I'm still healing a little bit more every day, although the burden I was carrying is getting lighter and lighter.

I have noticed periods of transition are especially likely to result in difficulty for me. In my case, I was transitioning to a different geographic location and professional endeavor. In my experience as a health coach, a majority of my clients were in some sort of life transition, be it in their work, relationships, or health.

Changes and transitions are inevitable, but how do we handle these transitions with respect to our identity? How do we tell our story to ourselves and others? How do we handle our past experiences, whether perceived as successes or failures, in the present and future?

Do we view past experiences that didn't go as well as we had hoped as failures?

It's important for people to build self-compassion and see past experiences—failures or successes—for what they are: learning experiences.

Self-Compassion: Don't Judge Yourself For Judging Yourself

I have come to believe that self-compassion is the single greatest untapped opportunity for our society to wake up and spread health, healing, and love to the world. In an effort to take my healing to the next level, I explored a lot of powerful books that helped deepen my relationship with myself. One of my favorites was *Self-Compassion: The Proven Power of Being Kind to Yourself* by Dr. Kristin Neff. Dr. Neff is one of the pioneers in exploring the role of intentional self-compassion in creating healing in our lives. In her book, Dr. Neff explains how to cultivate self-compassion:

> The only way to truly have compassion for yourself is to realize that your neurotic ego cycles are not your own choosing, they are natural and universal. Put simply, we come by our dysfunctions honestly—they are part of our human inheritance.

By reading Dr. Neff's book, I learned the value of not judging myself for judging myself.

You see, after my four-month modeling experience in Miami and some of the healing and learning that followed, I was still judging myself for the story I created in my mind:

> *TJ, how could you be so silly to focus so much on the physical. You know that's not what it's about. How could you be mystified by the glamour of the industry and let your ego get in the way?*

Judging ourselves about our past experiences only keeps us in a circle of judgment; a hamster wheel of suffering. Whatever the metaphor, this idea of judging ourselves for judging ourselves does not bring freedom, peace, or love. But having that awareness provides a great opportunity. A chance for us to choose acceptance for ourselves, our learning experiences, and even our "stories."

Instead of judging ourselves, or judging ourselves for judging ourselves, we can *choose* to look at our past experiences and our present relationship with ourselves through a lens of acceptance and compassion. If you're struggling with judging yourself for not being "good enough" in an area of your life, know that's alright. You are not alone, and you are exactly where you need to be. I accept you and invite you to do the same.

Over these last few years, I've processed and healed a lot from my past, especially my Miami modeling experience. It was as if this experience brought a lot of my unintegrated emotions (a.k.a. all my shit) up to the surface to see it transparently. And it provided me with an opportunity for so much beautiful growth rooted in choosing self-compassion.

Over the past seven years, working as a health coach, trainer, and consultant in the health and fitness community, so much energy and focus was placed on the physical. Nearly everyone I worked with had the goal of losing weight to look better and trying to improve their *physical* health.

And while I helped more and more people try to reach those same goals, I didn't realize I had lost focus on what is equally, if not more, important than our physical health—healing. Healing from the negative self-talk we put ourselves through. Healing from the stories we tell ourselves. And healing from placing so much energy on the physical.

I started to realize how an important part of achieving the health and performance we desire lies in our ability to be vulnerable. Igniting intentional vulnerability with courage and acceptance helped me share what was truly on my heart. And since then, I've experienced more freedom than I ever realized was possible. I have experienced a deeper level of my higher Self and released my ego along the way.

Through greater reflection, I realized that I didn't quite understand the power of what I now call the internal game of health—integrating the heart and spirit with the mind and body. In my case, my relationship with myself was rooted in the physical and mental parts of my body. I placed too much value on the external part of my health and only focused on what I thought were the healthiest habits: nutrition, fitness, and sleep.

As a health hacker, I was consumed by all of the *doing* to IMPROVE myself, that I lost sight of the importance of *being* and *feeling*. And most importantly, I lost sight of APPROVING of myself.

True health hackers look at their health holistically and find the right balance between APPROVING and IMPROVING their past and present Higher Selves.

Interestingly enough, da Vinci was the first person to discover that the heart, not the liver, was central to the blood system. Similarly, the heart is at the center of our approach to creating the most expansive, healthy, and fulfilling life possible.

Truth-Telling and Self-Expression

Whether we realize it or not, we all have stories we tell ourselves in our mind about our past, present, and future. And when considering the stories we tell ourselves, it's important to distinguish what's true and what's not true. While living in Miami, I had the pleasure of going through very powerful mastermind sessions led by my good friend, Phil Drolet, founder of The Feel Good Lifestyle. In these online and in-person sessions, we had the chance to learn some profound concepts that would help us build new skills and new ways of looking at the world. One of the topics that particularly resonated with me was the power of truth-telling.

During one of the online mastermind sessions, Drolet brought in his mentor and coach, Jesse Elder, for a powerful session called "The Four Levels of Truth-Telling." Elder described these four levels and everything started to shift for me. (*Note:* This is my interpretation of the four levels, and not specific definitions provided by anyone else.)

- **Level 1: Tell the Truth About Yourself To Yourself**

  If there's a habit or feature of your life you keep sweeping under the rug, think again. No need to lie to yourself *about yourself.* What good does that do? It's a protective mechanism that only limits us from our true potential and growth. At the same time, if you are telling yourself you are terrible or not good at something, realize you might be being a bit hard on yourself.

- **Level 2: Tell the Truth About Yourself to Others**

This is a true art of self-expression and is not easy. Be careful with what you express and to whom. But remember, we're all responsible for our own experience. You can't control how other people respond to your personal truth.

- **Level 3: Tell the Truth About Others to Yourself**

    If we're being honest, we tell stories to ourselves rooted in assumptions and judgments about others all the time. There is no need for that. This one is tricky, but if done right, can clear a lot of unnecessary mental and emotional anguish we tend to carry in our minds.

- **Level 4: Tell the Truth About Others to Others**

    This level of truth-telling requires an artful approach. Whether it's something "good" or "bad," it doesn't matter. Because it's not necessarily absolute truth; rather, it's *your* truth about someone else. It's still a story in your mind. But sharing that truth with others allows for clarity in conversations and a deepening relationship with whomever you are communicating, which can bring healing and human connection.

Each of these levels requires introspection as to how they relate to your life. And it doesn't come overnight. These levels can be applied to our present moment experiences as well as our past experiences. Here are some examples of these levels applied in my life.

Truth-Telling in My Life: My Relationship with Alcohol

When I returned to Iowa from my Miami modeling experience, my relationship with alcohol was not ideal. In Miami, I partied hard and developed a dependence on this substance to help me have fun. I fell into a vicious cycle of working out hard after a night of drinking, still trying to achieve the perfect body. I thought alcohol was harmless in small doses, but the problem was that the alcohol impacted several other areas of my life—my relationships with friends and family, as well as my relationship with food. Late nights of binge eating after even just a few drinks at a bar were part of the process for me.

Plus, as I got healthier and healthier, I became more and more sensitive to alcohol. Why? Because it's toxic! Or at least it has been for me.

About one month after I returned home to Iowa, I launched a 30-Day No Alcohol Challenge, inviting my friends to join me in giving up alcohol for a month. All in all, this was a big success. I had about thirty people go through the challenge with me. Most of us took intentional action and saw great results.

This was a big part of my growth and transition into my late twenties, and it started with telling the truth *to* myself, *about* myself.

There is no clear blueprint or proper environment for truthful authentic self-expression.

In fact, in the beginning, telling the truth can feel like driving an off-road vehicle through the woods toward authentic self-expression—a little bit scary and rugged. Just remember, the truth doesn't have to be pretty.

And when we muster up the courage to share our truth with others, it can bring a lot of peace and healing.

- What is your story?
- Have you told yourself the truth?
- Have you shared your truth with others?

If not, now is your chance to *choose yourself* in the most loving, self-compassionate way possible.

So many people in our country struggle with poor health and energy, and when you compound that with destructive thoughts and feelings, it can be a recipe for disaster.

I've learned it's natural for humans to want to grow, develop, and improve their lives; however, let's not undervalue the act of approving of ourselves along the way. Only after taking this important step—focusing on yourself, your story, and your heart—will you be ready to truly benefit from all that advancements in science and technology have to offer.

Summary:

- True health hackers look at their health holistically and find balance between approving and improving themselves.
- Judging ourselves for judging ourselves only keeps us in a hamster wheel of suffering. We have the opportunity to choose self-compassion at any time and in any moment.
- If you're struggling with judging yourself for not being "good enough" in an area of your life, that's OK. You're exactly where you need to be in this moment. I accept you and invite you to do the same.
- The Four Levels of Truth-Telling are powerful tools to help us get clear on how we communicate with ourselves and others.
- The truth doesn't have to be pretty. It just has to be true.

Action Items:

1. What's your story? And what stories are you telling yourself about your story? Could you use a little more self-compassion in your life?
2. Write a Letter To Yourself. Dr. Kristen Neff, author of *Self-Compassion: The Proven Power of Being Kind to Yourself*, provides an opportunity to communicate and relate to ourselves using a self-compassion letter-writing exercise:
   - Think of an aspect of your present-day self or a story about yourself from the past that you feel inadequate about. Maybe it's an area of your life where you don't feel like you're "good enough." Like me, maybe it has something to do with body image or your relationship with eating healthy foods. While you're holding onto this idea in your mind, start writing a letter to yourself from the perspective of an imaginary friend. Try to infuse your letter with as much love as possible.
   - To learn more about this exercise and Dr. Neff's work on self-compassion, visit her website: http://Self-Compassion.org.
3. Look at yourself in the mirror. Stare deeply into your eyes. Hug yourself and say, "I love you. I accept you. And I honor you for all the work you've put into this life." Then go find someone that you love, hug them, and tell them you love them.

ACT 2

The Rise of the Optimized:
Health Hackers Unite!

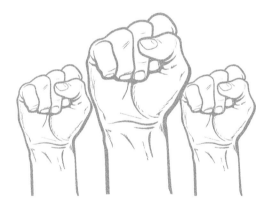

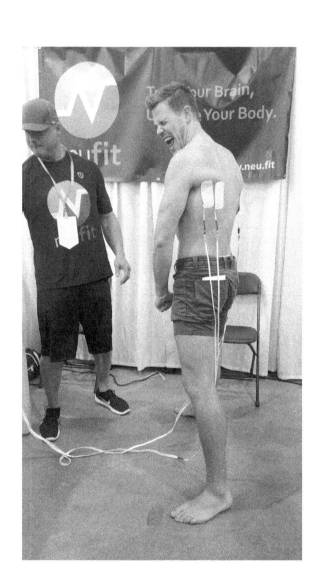

CHAPTER 4

_____

Hacking and Tracking Change Everything

*Not everything that counts can be counted and
not everything that can be counted counts.*
— ALBERT EINSTEIN

Over the past few decades, individuals and organizations have taken scientific and technological advancements to new heights, arguably quicker than any other time in human history. This rapid innovation has completely redefined how we as individuals use science, information, and technology to improve or "optimize" our overall health and performance. And the best part? The innovators behind these advancements are just getting started.

Take NeuFit out of Austin, Texas, for example. Founded by Garrett Salpeter, NeuFit may sound like just another gym or workout facility. On the contrary, using revolutionary, direct-current, electrical stimulation technology to help re-pattern the body's nervous system, NeuFit serves both the rehab market and fitness market in a completely different way.

I first met Salpeter and his team from NeuFit in spring 2016 at PaleoFx, one of the world's largest and most impressive health conferences held every year in Austin,

Texas. But it wasn't until later that year at the Bulletproof Biohacking Conference in Pasadena, California, that I realized what's possible with their machine.

Known as the NeuBie, NeuFit's high-powered direct-current electrical stimulation machine doesn't just find the pain points in your body, it helps to heal them. If you have experience in the physical therapy industry, you may have heard of a TENS machine that uses conventional electrical stimulation to provide short term symptom relief.

Similar to a TENS machine, the NeuBie uses electrical stimulation. But unlike most electrical stimulation machines, the NeuBie uses direct current, not alternating current. So instead of just providing short-term pain relief, the NeuBie provides deep healing to repattern the nervous system. Plus, by adding machine-assisted movement to the treatment, you're able to reprogram how the brain and body work together and optimize the nervous system.

NeuFit is an example of the powerful innovation happening to deliver next-level health and fitness outcomes to consumers. To receive this type of treatment, you would either need to go to Austin, Texas, or have a personal trainer or physical therapist in your area who owns a NeuBie and is trained in the NeuFit approach.

What other advancements are happening that can allow us to take action in our own health no matter where we live?

How else can we hack and track our health to bring about better outcomes in our own lives?

Let's start by taking a look at a popular movement known as the Quantified Self.

The Quantified Self

In fall 2010, Gary Wolf, journalist and editor for *Wired Magazine*, took the stage at TEDX Cannes with one simple, yet profound, message about our relationship with ourselves:

> The self is our operating center and moral compass. And if we want to act more effectively in the world, we have to get to know ourselves better.

He went on to share his personal tracking device data from the night before:

> I got up this morning at 6:10 a.m. after going to sleep at 12:45 a.m. I was awakened once during the night. My heart rate was sixty-one beats per minute. My blood pressure 127/74. I had zero minutes of exercise yesterday, so my maximum heart rate during exercise wasn't calculated. I had about six hundred milligrams of caffeine. Zero of alcohol. And my score on the narcissism personality index, or the NPI-16, is a reassuring 0.31.

The audience laughs and the ice is broken. Co-founder of the Quantified Self movement, Wolf is one of the pioneers in the use of self-tracking devices to gather information about oneself. His personal data from the night before provides a glimpse into how rapid advancements in technology are changing how we relate to ourselves, establish new habits, and make decisions that impact our health. Unless you've been under a rock for the past five or more years, you're probably aware of the uptick of self-tracking "wearable" devices being sold on the market. And you may even own one yourself.

CCS Insight, a global analysis company focused on mobile communications and the internet, predicts the wearables market will grow almost threefold by 2019, reaching an estimated 245 million wearable devices sold during that year. Furthermore, the wearables market will be worth $25 billion in 2019, with smartwatches predicted to account for nearly half of wearables revenue. We are witnessing and contributing to the advent of technology that brings us more data and information than we've ever had before. And as Wolf suggests, technology and the data it provides can serve as a way to know ourselves better:

> Now we know that new tools are changing our sense of self in the world. But we think of these tools as pointing outward, as windows. And I'd just like to invite you to think of them as turning inward, becoming mirrors. So we think of them as something to get a systematic improvement, we also think about how they can be useful for self-improvement, self-discovery, self-awareness, and self-knowledge.

Wolf's message is intriguing to say the least. During his talk he shared the technological factors driving the change in our lifestyles, including, the diffusion of mobile devices, exponential improvement in data storage and data processing, and remarkable improvements in biometric devices.

This is all great, but we need to make sure we're asking the right questions to manage how we relate to this movement. For example, what are the most important data to track to improve our health, energy, and life performance? And what type of data—qualitative or quantitative—should we be measuring? Should we be focusing all our energy on quantitative data, like hitting ten thousand steps or eating a certain number of calories per day? Or should we measure our metabolic resting heart rate and heart rate variability every morning and track how they change over time based on what we eat and drink, how we move, and the environments in which we spend our time?

There are a lot of different ways to measure the impact of different quantitative data we track throughout our lives, which we'll discuss throughout this book. But we also need to be mindful of qualitative data, like how we *feel* about an experience and how we make sense of the world. Either way, it's fair to say we now have the ability, more than ever before, to conduct our own experiments on ourselves and measure the quantitative and qualitative health impact of certain changes to our lifestyle and environment.

We'll discuss the Qualitative Self (QS) more in a bit, but first, we need to cover another important movement. As we approach new ways to improve ourselves and our health through data and technology, understanding the most basic scientific information about our biology is foundational to our success. Who are the leaders researching and applying these fundamental areas of health optimization?

Within the QS movement, there has been another movement of pioneers operating under the radar of mainstream health and wellness, waiting for the right moment to jump into the light. Well, it's safe to say they're out.

Enter the Biohackers

So what is a biohacker? A biohacker is similar to a computer hacker in that both are attempting to find a solution to a problem or gain control of a system. For a biohacker, the system being hacked is our human biology.

As I learned in a biohacking documentary episode of *SHIFT,* "Biohacking is almost as old as we are. As a species, we've been using technology to enhance our bodies for hundreds of thousands of years." We just haven't called it biohacking— until now.

Essentially, biohacking is a self-starting, alternative community made up of biohackers who use science and technology to make their bodies function better. And as with those involved in the QS movement, you better believe they like measuring their progress. For example, biohackers leverage the latest advanced lab testing to measure blood work, nutrient deficiencies, and genetic information. They focus on nutrition, exercise, proper hydration, and proper exposure to sunlight, as well as newer, more cutting-edge forms of optimizing our health and performance, like using nootropics, biometric devices, and even implanting electronic chips within the body.

Biohackers are doing amazing things to show us all how we are able to approach our self and improve our health.

Dr. Mark Ashton Smith, cognitive scientist from the Center for the Neural Basis of Cognition, believes the QS movement and biohackers are starting to come together:

> Biohacking has joined forces with the 'quantified self' movement resulting in a philosophy of self-experimentation and scientifically based training and technological intervention to improve human potential and performance.

At one time, this information was reserved for the smartest and most knowledgeable people in science and medical fields. Not anymore. In fact, many of the leading experts in today's health and biohacking space are self-starters who quit listening to the misinformation they were hearing about diet, for example.

I had the chance to interview Dave Asprey, creator of Bulletproof Coffee and author of *The Bulletproof Diet*, about his health journey and the biohacking movement overall. I had been following Asprey's Bulletproof blog and podcast for a while after a friend recommended I try his Bulletproof Coffee recipe. If you haven't heard of Bulletproof Coffee or wonder how it works, it involves blending healthy fats, like grass-fed butter and MCT Oil (highly concentrated coconut oil) into high-quality coffee, providing more sustainable energy and fewer crashes than if you used sugar or milk.

The Bulletproof movement is perhaps best known for its healthy, high-performance-inducing coffee cocktail, but the truth is, Bulletproof is about much more than coffee. It's one of the leaders in the next frontier of elevating the quality of our human experience and inspiring average consumers to learn more about their health. (Check out the top-rated health podcast, *Bulletproof Radio*, to learn more.)

Asprey, who refers to himself as a professional biohacker and is considered one of the pioneers of the biohacking movement, defines biohacking as "the art and science of changing the environment inside and outside your body so you have full control of your own biology." He was also a member of the Quantified Self movement, but became dissatisfied with just quantifying things—he wanted to change them. While talking about his story, he shared how changing his diet (from low fat to high fat) and his overall approach to health has made a positive impact on his life. "I lost 100 pounds. And I've kept it off for a long period of time," Asprey says. "Plus, I've turned my brain back on."

Asprey's success-story is an example of what's possible when we take our health into our own hands and track how our habits impact how we feel. He encourages others to follow in his footsteps by asking themselves the right questions:

> Carve your own path and ask yourself that question, like how am I feeling right now? How am I doing today? And better yet, measuring how you're doing. If you want to hack your biology measuring, what works is very important.

These are some of the fundamental questions leading biohackers, like Asprey, ask themselves on a daily basis. And this is the sort of self-coach approach we can use as well. Ultimately, Asprey's drastic health success was a result of him challenging the status quo of misinformation related to diet. Specifically, the notion that all calories are created equal and that fat is bad for us.

Thanks to advancements in science and technology over the past few years, this new group of health-conscious, quantified-self, biohacking humans are redefining how we approach our health and, perhaps, what it means to be human.

So how do we use the latest scientific advancements and knowledge in the most sustainable and effective way to improve and empower our health, instead of overwhelming us? We must remain keenly aware of how we relate to technology and how it impacts our state of health and performance.

The Downsides of Technology and Self-Tracking

Although we live in a world that uses technology to improve our lives, we must admit it has also changed how we relate to each other and ourselves. With this change comes the opportunity to know more about ourselves through data; however, data can also be overwhelming, and even misleading if we don't approach it in the right way. Technology can become addictive, and so can measuring our quantitative data.

For example, when I first experimented with a high fat ketogenic diet, I was measuring ketones in my breath and tracking that ketone data in a spreadsheet. (Ketones are an alternative energy source to glucose that result from a ketogenic diet high in healthy fat, moderate protein, and very low carbohydrates and sugar. More on that later.) For a brief period, it was interesting to measure how my ketone levels played a role in my physical and mental performance, but after a few weeks, I became overwhelmed with knowing every exact ketone level. It was becoming more of a time waster for me. And that's OK; it wasn't essential to my health. I felt the mental and physical benefits from eating a higher fat diet and I didn't need to measure every single metric.

Some people have started to write and talk about the over-quantified self— the person who feels overwhelmed by managing all sorts of health data and the very act of measuring one's health leads to more unnecessary stress.

With the number of people interested in using technology to track, measure, and learn more about themselves at an all-time high, the question we ought to be asking ourselves is this: How do we use technology to empower, not limit, ourselves and our quest for health optimization?

I hope we can all agree that striking a balance between our use of technology, our understanding and application of science, and the information we generate from ourselves requires an intentional, artful approach.

Enter The Qualitative Self

The concept of the Qualitative Self is focused on the aspects of our being that we cannot count or measure. The Qualitative Self is, in essence, self-awareness through reflection. It is characterized by feedback loops that involve our hearts and our minds to reflect on and learn from our experiences, perhaps providing an added sense of health, well-being, and purpose. It's one thing to have data and information about your body, and another thing to simply know how you feel.

Put another way, we must make sure we don't get caught up in measuring every little detail of our health while ignoring how we feel about our experience.

Einstein was right when he said, "Not everything that counts can be counted and not everything that can be counted counts."

You can buy several different wearables to track your movement, sleep, and other biomarkers like resting heart rate and blood pressure. Alternatively, you can save your money and focus your efforts on journaling about your symptoms and feelings to track how often you are sick or why you might be feeling bad.

Health data are not the finish line, they are the starting block. We need to make sure the simple delivery of health data is not seen as the solution, but rather the first step to making our health data relevant and actionable.

As discussed in chapter 2, reaching optimized health requires an integrated approach. It truly is the integration between our thoughts, feelings, and behaviors that allows us to develop into complete, whole, and healthy humans. Data allow us to learn about ourselves, but those data are not helpful unless we can make sense of them and take appropriate action that improves the quality of our life experience.

It's true—hacking and tracking has changed everything. It's our job to manage this change in a sustainable, optimized, and intentional way.

Summary:

- The Quantitative Self and Biohacking movements are democratizing health optimization and self-improvement to the average consumer by minimizing assumptions and empowering self-experimentation with respect to our health.
- The concept of the Qualitative Self is an opportunity to look beyond measurable data and look into our feelings and awareness.
- We don't lack the science, information, or technology to live healthy. We lack the art to know how to use them properly.
- Health optimization requires a balance between measuring and monitoring our Quantitative Self (how we measure and reflect on data that can be counted, like body fat percentage and heart rate) and our Qualitative Self (how we feel about our experience).
- You can buy several different wearables to track your movement, sleep, and other biomarkers. Alternatively, you can save your money and focus your efforts on journaling about your symptoms and feelings.

Action Items:

1. What quantitative information do you currently track about yourself or your health (e.g., daily steps with your wearable tracking device, hours slept, workouts per week, calories per day)?
   - What have you learned about yourself as a result of tracking this information?
   - Do you feel like tracking this data is useful? Do you think this is the most important health information to track?

2. What qualitative information do you use to check in with yourself?
   - How do you feel in the morning, afternoon, or evening?
   - How do you feel after you eat a certain food?

3. What areas of your health may be helpful to measure in the future? If you're new to measuring your progress in these ways, spend seven days adding some intention to how you measure and monitor both your quantitative and qualitative metrics and see what you learn.

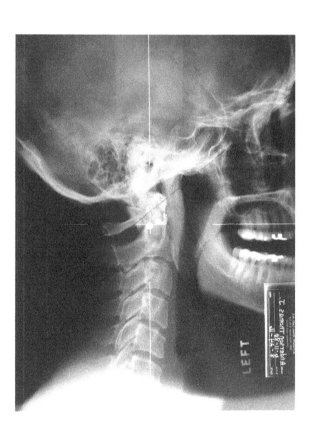

CHAPTER 5

What is Health Hacking?

*Every patient is an expert in their own chosen field, namely
themselves and their own life.*
– Emma Hill

As we have discussed, the traditional US health care system is changing, but not at the rate of some other health-related movements. The hackers and trackers are changing how we can reclaim our personal health outside of the traditional health care system as we know it.

Who are Health Hackers?

Health hackers are individuals who consciously take their health into their own hands by researching the most up-to-date science and, most of all, experimenting with new and intentional behaviors, habits, and routines.

And what is (the art of) Health Hacking, exactly?

Health hacking is an efficient and effective self-coach approach to reaching the optimal, holistic health and sustainable performance one desires. Think of health hacking as a creative shortcut to optimizing your health as well as feeling and performing your best. It's a mindset, it's a practice, and it's a way of life.

I came up with the title of this book, *The Art of Health Hacking*, after being inspired by the biohacking movement through my work in health coaching, both inside and outside of the traditional health care system. But at the time, biohacking did not completely resonate with me. It seemed to be filled with a lot of scientific information that was a bit overwhelming. Plus, if you Google "biohacking" you'll likely stumble upon several videos and articles about the technical side of biohacking (e.g., transhumanism, futurism, and singularity) and the concept of augmenting or upgrading the human experience. Don't get me wrong, those movements are exciting and interesting to think about, but I wanted to write a book to help build a bridge between those who are generally interested in their health and those who are operating with peak health, energy, and performance.

And so the creative health coach in me started to fall in love with the concept of health hacking, and becoming a health hacker myself. I wanted to make these health concepts more accessible to the average health-conscious consumer by answering a few important questions:

- What are the fundamentals of reaching health optimization?
- What are the greatest opportunities for a personal health revolution in this country?
- How can we, as true health hackers, unite in a cohesive, uplifting manner?
- Could we build a whole new model of health care characterized by high-quality, holistic health care teams and self-care strategies rooted in disease prevention, personal health empowerment, and radical self-care?

It involves going down the rabbit hole to realize how much is possible in our health, and when you get there, to understand that no matter where you currently are on the health spectrum, developing a more artful, creative approach to intentional and sustainable action is the key to our success.

This chapter will describe the unique rise in those who are reaching a new level of optimization—the health hackers.

Before we go any further, let's clear something up. The term "hacker" can be viewed negatively in our culture, conjuring stories of stealing personal information online. But when I refer to "hackers" throughout this book, I mean it in a positive way. As a review, here is how I define **holistic health hackers:**

> Holistic health hackers are individuals who view their health as interconnected parts that make up a whole. Holistic health hackers are proactive (not reactive), and ultimately take their health into their own hands as much as possible. They are ready to learn and take action when appropriate and also reflect on their experiences.

In this chapter, we're going to be learning and understanding more about our own personal health data. Health hacking does not aim to overwhelm you with tons of information. Rather, it's an actionable approach aimed at simplifying your focus and optimizing your outcomes—how you feel and perform.

Health hacking is the act of doing health. That is, combining clever health hacks into the personal process of sustainable health optimization. My definition of health hacking is based on how I view health, and I invite you to try it on for size in your own life. Some people want to know all the biological pathways involved when making a specific nutrition or lifestyle change, and understanding how those principles relate to health is important to them. In contrast, some people don't like to get too quantitative or scientific with their health, preferring to focus on things that are more understandable, applicable, and relevant. But remember, health hacking can be whatever you want it to be.

When you really start to think about your health, it can feel overwhelming. Let's begin by considering some powerful principles to use when approaching your health.

The 5 Ps of Health Hacking

1. Preparation

Being mindful of our health as we prepare for our day can make such a big difference in how our day actually unfolds. Whether it's preparing your meals in advance, packing a bag for the gym, traveling with a lacrosse ball to roll out your muscles on a business trip, or simply scheduling moments in your day for a mindfulness break, setting the intention to be mindful of your health can make a world of difference. Not only does it allow you to prepare for what you want (or have) to do, but also *who* and *what* you desire to be.

2. Prevention

As we have discussed, so much sickness and disease is preventable. It's also important to realize that feeling sluggish and worn out throughout the day is also preventable. We make healthy decisions because we want to feel good in the present, and also prevent feeling bad in the future.

3. Performance

Health hacking is about creating what's possible in our health so we are in a position to create the "impossible" in our life. Our health sets the stage for our ability to perform to the best of our ability. Our health impacts how we perform in our work, relationships, and every area of our life. Realizing and remembering this principle can bring clarity and focus to the *why* of what we are doing to improve and maintain our health. Our health can truly be an asset in our work and relationships.

4. Progress

Health hacking is an active approach. It is all about the journey, not the destination. Celebrating progress throughout our health optimization journey is vital to our continued motivation, interest, and success. When we reach a goal or complete a habit—great! Let's give ourselves some credit and celebrate our progress.

5. Presence

Last, but certainly not least, health hacking involves creating and maintaining presence in our everyday lives. Maintaining presence in our bodies and our minds allows us to go about our day in a peaceful and effortless way. Presence is living in the now. And it just may be the single most important principle of the 5 Ps of Health Hacking. We'll dive into how we can cultivate more present moment awareness later on in the book.

Now that we know a little bit more about what health hacking can mean, let's take a look at what health hacking is not.

What Health Hacking is Not

When we look to improve our health, it is important to remember that we are human. And our perfection can be found in our imperfection. In fact, developing a perfection mindset on our health hacking journey can be one of the main causes of problems when it comes to seeing improvement. The intention is to learn and grow, while finding an optimal outcome—aiming for progress, not perfection.

How do we keep our focus on "good enough," or set an intention to live with optimal, rather than perfect, health? The perfection mindset is not something that goes away easily. It is real and must be addressed. While directing a lot of time and energy to my modeling experience, I became overly focused on achieving what my agents would call a "tighter body." I wanted to achieve 8 percent body fat. I wanted to look good for the cameras, and if I didn't, I felt like a failure. I used to think a perfection mindset only applied to my experience with the physical body, but I have realized that this perfection mindset does not start or end with the physical. The perfection mindset can be better understood within the context of the following four areas of health:

The Physical Body–How We Look in the Mirror

Our physical health is much more than how we look. More importantly, it's about how you feel and function in your everyday life. Focusing only on your looks can lead to unhealthy thought patterns and feelings of not being "good enough."

The Mental Body–How We Relate to our Thoughts

We can also develop a perfection mindset toward the types of thoughts we have and how well we are able to perform certain mental functions (e.g., focus or memory). You are not your thoughts. You are more than your ability to think perfectly.

The Emotional Body–How We Feel

Striving for the goal of feeling perfect all of the time can also be an unhealthy mindset. It's OK to be stressed every now and then. It's OK to not feel as energized or as happy as we would like. It is during these times that we can feel gratitude for the times we *do* feel energized and in control of our health.

Our Actions and Behaviors–What we are doing, what we want to do, and who we want to be

Having a perfectionist approach toward our actual habits and behaviors can be unhealthy as well. It's great to focus on making healthy decisions, but it's OK not to visit the gym or yoga mat every day. It's OK that you ate ice cream, chocolate, or pizza.

Remember, health hacking is not about perfection. It's about being open to learning about and striving for health optimization. Seeking perfection in our thoughts, our feelings, and our actions is a trap we can all fall into on any given day. Sometimes it seems that is how we are hardwired to think. It's important to acknowledge these thoughts, feelings, and behaviors for what they are—an interest in improving ourselves and being good enough in our own eyes and the eyes of others. Remember that it takes a different way of thinking to *approve* of ourselves where we are today.

The truth is, we're already perfect as we are going to be, right now in this moment.

Health Literacy

Another way to look at health optimization is the idea of being successful in one's health. According to the US Department of Health and Human Services, the term **health literacy** is used to describe one's "capacity to obtain, process, and understand basic health information and services needed to make appropriate health decisions."

You'll notice that this definition does not include the act of performing healthy behaviors or making actual decisions. Health literacy applies more to our *capacity to make decisions* and take actions that will lead to desired outcomes.

We must understand that in order for us to make appropriate, healthy decisions and reach desired outcomes, we must first make a commitment to advancing our own health literacy.

Become a Self Expert, not a Health Expert

When I started becoming more passionate about health, I learned a lot about health, the human body, and behavior change. Often this information was represented as absolute truth: the human body works in a certain way. However, the more I read and learned, the more I realized there are very few absolute truths and so much gray area. That is when I decided that I was not going to try to become a scientific genius or health expert. I was going to seek more health literacy and less perfection. I believe this is where we have an opportunity to change the way we see and relate to our health. Instead of feeling overwhelmed by health information, I invite you to see your health as a hobby.

See Your Health as a Hobby

Most of you reading this book right now are adults interested in learning a thing or two about your health. So how do adults learn? By developing a willingness to admit they don't know something, sometimes followed by an interest in developing a new hobby based on what they learned.

Think about some of your hobbies. Maybe you're a reader, writer, painter, dancer, or climber. Whatever your interests, I'm guessing you have come to enjoy those activities after developing a willingness to learn and a commitment to action. A hobby is something we do in our spare time for fun. It's not our full-time job and it doesn't have to be. It's something we can engage in on the side because we enjoy it and it improves our quality of life.

The same can be said of our health. If we start looking at our health as a hobby, a lot can change. Our entire approach, including how we learn and take action with respect to food intake, nutrition, movement, and sleep, can allow our health to unfold in an effortless and artful way.

Now this is where people may start to get in their heads a bit and say, "But that's my issue! I have no time!"

First, I understand. Time is a precious resource. And lack of time is one of the most common objections or excuses people provide when talking about their health (e.g., shopping for health food, preparing food, working out). In the Action Items section at the end of this chapter, you'll have an opportunity to complete a time-management exercise to take a good look at where you are spending your time. (*Hint:* it has a lot to do with getting creative and identifying your priorities.)

Have you ever thought of your health as a hobby? Either way, there is an opportunity to realize that health doesn't have to be hard. On the contrary, our health is something we can take pleasure in. We can see focusing on our health as a time for us to engage in behaviors we enjoy that also support our health. I think it's time we start viewing health as a hobby and make it fun again!

We will strive for optimal health, not perfect health. And we'll have plenty of fun along the way.

This is your chance to become a health hacker, commit to growing your health literacy, and view the pursuit of your health as a hobby.

Summary:

- **Health hacking is an efficient and effective self-coach approach toward reaching the optimal health and performance you desire.**
- Health Hacking is not about perfection. It's OK to have perfectionist thoughts and an interest in improvement, but remember that we're on a journey toward sustainable health optimization—not perfection.
- Remember the 5 Ps of Health Hacking: Preparation, Prevention, Performance, Progress, and Presence.
- Health Hacking is not about becoming a health expert, but a self expert.
- Viewing health as a hobby and developing a willingness to learn new things can influence how we think about and take action in pursuit of health.

Action Items:

1. Review the 5 Ps of Health Hacking (Preparation, Prevention, Performance, Progress, and Presence).

    - If you find it helpful, consider texting, e-mailing, or talking to a friend or family member about one or more of the 5 Ps of Health Hacking.

    - Then read them out loud. As you say each word out loud, pause, and let them sink into your soul. Notice what comes up for you. Ask yourself, "How do I feel when I hear that word?" Did something come up in your body or mind as you thought about one or more of the 5 Ps of Health Hacking?

    - Reflect. How did you feel about this exercise? What did you learn about yourself in this chapter? What resonated with you in particular?

2. Time-Management Exercise

    - Take a piece of paper and divide it into four quadrants by drawing a large cross. Label the top left quadrant "Start Doing," the top right quadrant "Stop Doing," the bottom left quadrant "Do More Of," and the bottom right quadrant "Do Less Of."

    - Now take a moment to think about all of the activities that fill your day, from morning to night. Begin to fill each quadrant with the activities that fit each description. What activities would you like to start doing, stop doing, do more of, or do less of?

    - By consciously deciding to spend more of your time doing the things you want to be doing and less of your time doing the things you don't want to be doing, you may actually have the power to "create" more time in your day.

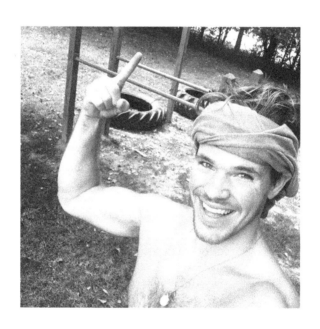

CHAPTER 6

From Health Coaching to Self Coaching:

It Starts with a Question

Change is not an event, it's a process.
– Cheryl James

If this new sense of empowerment through health hacking is to improve our health, where do we go from here? It's time we delve into the science and art of sustainable behavior change and examine the power of health coaching and its role in self coaching.

Don't "Should" On Me

When I meet someone new and they ask what I do for a living or what I am passionate about, they seem intrigued when I answer, "health coaching for behavior change."

Then they might ask what they're doing wrong in their health or if a specific type of food or workout is truly "healthy." If I'm really lucky, they may ask some deeper questions: "Health coaching? What exactly does that mean? Do you just tell people what they **should** eat or what workouts they should do?" I usually answer something like this: "Well, not exactly. Personally, I don't like being "should" on. Let's face it—that can get pretty messy. So I usually don't "should" on others; unless they want me to."

Poop jokes and laughter ensue.

In today's world, we use the word *should* more often than we—should. (Oops!) It's true. We project our beliefs and opinions on others in a way that limits their ability to discover something on their own. This word is particularly overused in our conversations related to health—what we deem as living healthy. The result? The person does not follow through or own the ideas being presented because they are being *told* what they should do.

And if we're honest, we probably do this to others and ourselves more than we'd like to admit.

To illustrate this point, here are some examples of well-meaning friends, family, or colleagues telling someone else what they *should* do:

Scenario 1: You're in a group of friends and you start talking about how you want to start working out again. Maybe it's been several weeks or months and you recognize this is an area in which you need to take action. All of a sudden, a friend leans over to you and says, "You *should* really be lifting weights. Here's this great fitness program to follow. It's such a great workout—you'll feel amazing!"

After taking several weeks or even months off of working out, how would you feel after someone told you what you *should* be doing?

Scenario 2: Consider nutrition—a very personal topic in the world of health. Since you're reading this book I'm guessing you've started to take an interest in ways you can improve what you eat.

How would it feel if someone told you that you should or should not be eating a certain food or a certain way?

Would that comment leave you with positive feelings, as if they just helped you solve a problem? Or would you be turned off by them telling you what you *should* be doing?

I'm guessing you would be turned off. But it depends on how open you are. I'll be the first to admit I used to do this. After researching and experimenting with something that was beneficial to me, I developed a belief about it, and wanted to share it with the world. After experiencing success in one area of my life (e.g., getting in shape, improving how I felt), it seemed I couldn't help but share it with the world.

Did either of these "should" scenarios sound familiar to you? Have you ever been the person being told what they should do? Have you ever been the person telling others what they should do? Maybe both? We may not be conscious of it while it's happening, but it can lead to a potentially stressful conversation with whomever you're speaking. This approach may stem from someone's excitement about a personal experience or recent revelation in their own life; however, it's not always well-received. Especially if you (or they) have already been making an effort to improve other areas of health.

According to leading memory and learning expert Jim Kwik, "Your mind is always eavesdropping on your self-talk." So take inventory of the words you say to yourself— spoken or not—as you consider changing a behavior.

We can change how we communicate with each other and ourselves in a way that makes life easier, supports understanding and clarity, and helps people build stronger, more meaningful relationships.

How is Health Coaching different?

The truth is, health coaching is all about asking simple, yet powerful, questions.

The mission of the properly trained health coach is to empower someone to be the leader in their own health. Health coaches don't focus on teaching and telling; they are trained to use specific skills to ask, listen, and inspire someone to take action in a sustainable, empowered way. Health coaches co-create a plan of action with clients to build healthier habits, and in turn, increase their clients' focus, productivity, and peace of mind.

Don't get me wrong. Understanding the actual details of what foods to eat and workouts to do is hugely important. In fact, this is one of the main areas that sets great health coaches apart from average health coaches. A great health coach knows when to share certain information and resources and when to just listen.

Understanding and properly applying the fundamentals of nutrition in our lives is important. But sometimes it requires an artful approach—a different way to go about it. Because health is so much more than diet and fitness.

Our health isn't just poor because of poor nutrition education, big food companies, and limited access to healthy foods. Our health starts with developing deep, loving, personal relationships with others as well as ourselves. That's what health coaching and self coaching can provide.

This chapter will introduce several key health coaching principles with the hope that you will experiment with these methods of communicating with yourself about your health, and as a "buddy coach" to friends, colleagues, family members, or clients.

You can also apply these principles when hiring a health coach. Because having someone who is trained in and has experience utilizing the highest level of conscious health coaching communication can elevate you to sustainable and intentional action.

The Number One Key to Health Coaching: Communication

Before I got into health coaching, I had no idea how powerful communication skills were in supporting people to improve their health. Fast-forward to the present day, and I've realized it's one of the biggest game changers—not just in the world of formal health care, but in our relationship with ourselves, our friends, and our families. I believe that's where true health care actually occurs: in our relationships with ourselves and everyone around us. If we can support the creation of relationship transformation, we're onto something powerful that can truly turn health care on its head.

Before we dive deeper into transforming how we communicate with each other, let's take another look into our health care system today. While we have discussed the idea of building an entirely new model outside of our traditional health care system, there is still a thing or two to learn about the current model to provide some context.

Patient Education Inside the System

If you look at health care today, most health professionals went through years of schooling to become experts at fixing the broken and healing the sick. But most were not taught two key elements:

- The power to promote sustainable behavior change through conscious health coaching conversations
- The power to provide support and education on functional, lifestyle, and preventative health topics such as nutrition, exercise, and stress management

And it's this combination of proper coaching and effective teaching that can yield the most powerful results.

In health care, there is a tremendous focus on patient education. I have had many conversations with health care professionals about their efforts to teach and educate patients.

It's one of the guiding principles health systems have used for the past several decades to try to get patients to change. But there's a problem. Patient education doesn't work most of the time. Think about it for a moment. If you're eating a diet high in sugar and processed foods, consuming too much alcohol or tobacco, or hardly working out, most likely you already know that these behaviors are not very healthy. Most humans have a certain amount of common sense about what's healthy and what's not, but that doesn't necessarily mean they are willing or able to change—on their own.

That's why patient education falls short. We can't just teach people—especially adults—who aren't necessarily interested in learning. Adult education doesn't work that way. There must be a willingness to learn.

In my experience, that willingness to learn and the behavior change process is different for everyone and requires patience, empathy, and a new, skillful way of communicating. Over the past few years, both inside and outside of traditional health care settings, these conversations have been happening, thanks in part to a surge in the popularity of health coaching.

Health Coaching in Health Care: A Skill Set, Not Just a Profession

Imagine if you could learn and develop conscious communication skills that would allow you to ask the right questions and listen to yourself so you can make stress-free, highly aligned, healthy decisions as well as develop the capacity to help others in your life do the same. These represent some of the most important skills health coaching professionals use.

Now imagine if we could democratize these skill sets, so individuals could not just learn how to coach and guide themselves, but also coach and guide the friends, family, and colleagues they care about most.

Health coaching is not just a profession. It's a skill set. But it's a skill set that doesn't have to be limited to a formal setting. Health coaching skills can be learned and used by all to improve how we communicate and relate to each other.

So what does health coaching actually entail?

There are many different health coach training programs available. I spent two years leading business development for one of them: the Clinical Health Coach. This is one of the most powerful trainings I've seen integrate key communication skills related to Motivational Interviewing and the Transtheoretical Model of Behavior Change, among others.

There are also a few powerful coaching technology platforms available today that connect consumers with a health coach or care provider in a dynamic and user-friendly way, including Nudge, Coach.Me, and Twine. If you're a health coach or health professional interested in improving your effectiveness with patients, I suggest you look into these platforms.

But what about consumers? What do they think about these apps and health coaching in general?

In an April 2016 survey, Twine Health asked five hundred US adults about their interest in and knowledge and awareness of health coaching. The results were surprising: 60 percent of respondents were interested in receiving health coaching, 80 percent had never been offered health coaching, and 60 percent preferred digital health coaching (versus 22 percent who preferred receiving health coaching over the telephone).

While these results don't tell the whole story, they do paint a picture of the general public's experience of health coaching.

Now you may be wondering, how does someone learn something new about their health if the other person is only asking questions? That's where asking for permission to share comes into play. Health coaches can take off their proverbial "coach hat" and ask permission to put on their "consultant hat" to share something if they believe it will make a big difference for the other person.

You may also question the abilities or legitimacy of a health coach, because some health coaches aren't licensed medical professionals. But Dr. Roger Jahnke, chief executive officer of the consulting and training firm Health Action believes otherwise. "People with medical degrees think about health intervention," says Jahnke. "It's an illusion that medicine is prevention—it's intervention. Prevention is people taking care themselves. The coach is there to support a person making a reasonable plan."

It's really all about co-creating a plan for sustainable behavior change; however, it's important to note that this plan is not a one-size-fits-all approach. It's all customizable and specific to the patient or client involved.

Have you ever felt rushed to change a habit? Maybe you weren't totally ready to make a change, but someone was rushing you into something? If so, you're not alone. In fact, a lot of people mistakenly start a new habit when they're not quite ready.

The truth is, we all may have a list of habits we want to pick up. There are several areas of our health we may want to focus on, but we may not be ready to start making changes in every one of those areas all at once. It requires patience to move through the stages of behavior change. To help you understand how this all works, here is a quick overview of what is referred to as the Transtheoretical Model of Behavior Change.

The Transtheoretical Model of Behavior Change

The Transtheoretical Model (TTM) of Behavior Change, also known as the Stages of Change, is one of the leading models of behavior change used by professionals worldwide. Originally developed by James O. Prochaska and Carlo

DiClemente in 1983, the Transtheoretical Model is an integrative, biopsychosocial model that conceptualizes the process of intentional behavior change.

Dr. Prochaska went on to found Pro-Change Behavior Systems Inc., an internationally recognized behavior change company that offers evidence-based health and wellness solutions to reduce health risk behaviors, maximize well-being, lower health care costs, and increase productivity.

According to the Pro-Change website, other models of behavior change focus exclusively on certain dimensions of change (social or biological influences), whereas the TTM seeks to include and integrate key elements from other theories into a comprehensive theory of change (hence the name Transtheoretical) that can be applied to a variety of behaviors, populations, and settings.

Based on principles developed from over forty years of scientific research, intervention development, and a plethora of empirical studies, the TTM is the theoretical basis for a lot of health coach trainings and provides a framework for both professionals and consumers to understand how the behavior change process unfolds over time.

Five Stages of Change

Here are the five stages of change and a description of each:

1. **Precontemplation** (Not Ready): Not intending to change this behavior
2. **Contemplation** (Getting Ready): Intending to make this behavior change in the next six months
3. **Preparation** (Ready): Intending to make this behavior change in the next thirty days
4. **Action**: Have been engaging in the new behavior for less than six months
5. **Maintenance**: Have been engaging in the new behavior for more than six months

A lot of people want know how long it takes to build a new habit, and according to this model of behavior change, six months is a general benchmark for a person to fully integrate a habit. It doesn't have to be strictly six months, so remember this—only *you* know what phase you are in at any given time for a particular habit.

The behaviors I shared earlier (e.g., smoking, drinking alcohol, poor diet, lack of movement) are just some of the key behaviors driving the chronic disease epidemic in our country. You may or may not exhibit these particular behaviors, but I'm guessing you can think of a few behaviors that you would consider changing to improve your overall health.

But before you do, let's take a look at another powerful process for navigating behavior change—conscious communication. The most effective health coaches and health coach training organizations include a strong motivational interviewing component, utilizing strategies such as reflective listening and open-ended questions.

Motivational Interviewing

Motivational Interviewing is a well-known behavior change communication strategy. In fact, **Motivational Interviewing is one of the most evidence-based strategies for encouraging behavior change in health care.** At Clinical Health Coach, we trained a few thousand health care professionals across the country in this method of communicating. The goal? To help them transform conversations with patients to encourage sustainable behavior change—where the patient feels empowered and activated to take some sort of action in their own health.

There are a lot of components involved in Motivational Interviewing. While it is beyond the scope of this book to share everything I've learned about Motivational Interviewing, I want to give you a taste of what's possible when you integrate some of these concepts of health coaching into your life.

Motivational Interviewing requires a fair amount of training and practice; however, in the book *Motivational Interviewing: Helping People Change*, authors Rollnick and Miller break down this concept into an easy-to-understand acronym: O.A.R.S.

Defining O.A.R.S.

O–Open-ended Questions

- Open-ended questions are those questions that you cannot answer with a "yes" or "no" response. Unlike a closed-ended question, open-ended questions require more of a thoughtful response.
  - For example, if you're communicating with yourself (or someone else) about a habit you (or they) want to start or stop, an opened-ended question may be, "What makes you feel it might be time for a change?"
- Although closed-ended questions are sometime necessary and useful, open-ended questions are a great way to create forward momentum in our quest to help ourselves and others explore behavior change.

A–Affirmation

- Affirmations are statements of recognition about someone's particular strength, and are typically suggested to be used in areas where we normally perceive failure. Our minds tend to focus on the negative. It's a cognitive bias we all have. In order to support our ability to focus on the positive, it's important for us to recognize our own skills and strengths as well as the skills and strengths of others.
- For example, if you recently got off track with a new workout routine and are getting down on yourself, you could incorporate both affirmations and open-ended questions by saying to yourself, **"You worked out for a week successfully. How were you able to stay committed to working out that week?"**
- Do you see how that question is worded in an affirming, positive way? We're not running from the value of learning from our mistakes, rather we're staying focused on how we can learn from and follow our patterns of success.

R-Reflective Listening

- Listening is demonstrated in three ways: not interrupting, responding to what the person is saying, and reflecting back to deepen the conversation.
- Reflective listening is the golden key to unlocking the beauty of health coaching and self coaching. If we're able to cultivate better listening skills with ourselves and others, we'll all feel a lot more heard, understood, appreciated, and confident in ourselves and our ability to move forward.
- Reflective listening is truly an art. It is not about asking questions, but reflecting back what you heard in statements. It can be simply repeating or rephrasing what you heard, or can be more complex (e.g., add meaning, use metaphors, incorporate emotion or importance). Typically, your voice goes down at the end of each statement.
- Here are some examples of how you can start a reflective statement as a part of your reflective listening.
  - If someone expresses an interest in eating healthier, but doesn't know where to start, you could respond with, "It sounds like you have an interest in choosing healthier foods to eat and you might know a few ways to do so, but you're unsure of where to begin."

S-Summaries

- Summaries reinforce the language of "change talk" (language you hear yourself or others use when talking about something they're interested in changing) as a powerful tool to help transition a person into planning mode.
- For example, if you're finishing a conversation with yourself (or others) about your interest in changing a habit, make sure you summarize the conversation to transition into planning the habits you want to start changing.

As you can see, health coaching uses a mode of communication that anyone can learn and add to their arsenal. Yes, nurses, doctors, nutritionists, personal trainers, and many other health professionals could benefit from transforming how they communicate with each other, and especially with patients and clients.

But so can the general public. You and I can become health coaches for ourselves and others, guiding and empowering each other to create sustainable behavior change.

Imagine having the skills to coach yourself and others—like friends, family, and colleagues—by listening and communicating in the most powerful way possible. The result? You could hold space for people on a whole new level, accepting them where they are now and supporting them however they want or need to be supported. We're talking next level personal health empowerment. And activation.

Raj Lahoti, a wise man and personal mentor of mine once said, **"Smart people have answers. Geniuses have questions."** And contrary to popular belief, genius status is no longer relegated to a special few. We all have the power to be geniuses in our own life, in our own way.

For more than seven years, I've worked in and around the health care system learning how hospitals, clinics, and health professionals support patients to improve their health. It's baffling how many challenges must be overcome to actually make a difference through sustainable behavior change.

But if we, as friends, families, and colleagues, all unite as true health hackers to support each other with conscious conversations outside the traditional health care system, I believe we can make a meaningful difference. Remember—health coaching and self coaching begin with a single question and end with intentional listening.

Summary:
- Don't "should" on others (or yourself!). How we communicate is a choice and a skill requiring practice and intention.
- Health coaching is not just a profession, but a skill set we can all learn. It starts with a question and ends with powerful listening skills.
- Change requires patience; it doesn't happen overnight. According to the Transtheoretical Model (TTM) of Behavior Change, there are actually five stages of change we pass through as we consider a new habit or behavior: Precontemplation, Contemplation, Preparation, Action, and Maintenance.

- **O.A.R.S.** stands for:
  - **Open-ended questions** are received better than closed-ended questions, with ourselves and others.
  - **Affirmations** help you focus on and feel empowered to replicate the positive—not to run away from the negative.
  - **Reflections** help someone feel not just listened to, but genuinely heard—there is a difference.
  - **Summaries** help you emphasize "change talk" to encourage transition into planning mode.
- "Smart people have answers. Geniuses have questions." –Raj Lahoti

Action Items:

1. How do you currently approach behavior change or manage your interest in changing habits?
2. In what areas of your health are you in precontemplation or contemplation mode?
3. How do you communicate with yourself? Do you journal? Do you ask yourself questions? If so, do you ask open-ended questions or closed-ended questions?
4. Do you engage in negative self-talk? If so, how do you handle it?
5. Ask your friends how they experience your communication skills. Ask permission to share what you've learned in this chapter.
6. Find a Coaching Buddy. Use what you've learned in this chapter about health coaching and find people to practice with. This could be a good friend, family member, or an acquaintance. Don't just choose one—experiment with a few. It's important to note the intention of these conversations (with ourselves and others) is not necessarily to force behavior change and goal setting, but rather to establish clarity around potential goals one may have interest in acting on.
7. **BONUS:** My Ultimate, Present-Moment HACKronym.

   As we've discussed, this is a book about coaching ourselves in our own health. To help remind ourselves of the power of coaching ourselves and what it actually means to coach ourselves, I created this acronym:

C.O.A.C.H.
Choose This Moment…and Breathe
Observe Your Experience…and Feel
Assess Your Stress…and Heal
Communicate with Clarity…and Trust
Have Fun and Smile

Take the time to go through each step, one by one, until you finally get to FUN. And then you can realize what's possible with this unique, self-coach approach.

ACT 3

Behind the Scenes:

The Inner Game of Health and Healing

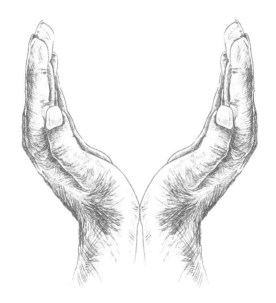

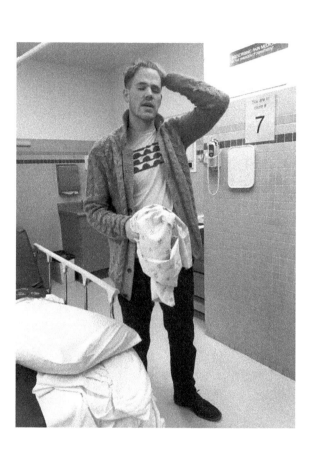

CHAPTER 7

Create Clarity:

Get Real With How You Feel

*"During this journey, our intention is not to attempt
to feel good, but rather to feel real."*
– MICHAEL BROWN

Have you ever been at a point in your life where you felt a bit overwhelmed or stressed out?

Maybe you were in the process of juggling responsibilities at work or thinking about all of the areas of your health that you need to get right. Or maybe you've had moments of wanting to get clear on where you stand in your life—who you are, how healthy and happy you are, or what you want to create in the world.

If so, keep reading. We're going to peel back the curtains and take a look at what's really going on behind the scenes of our health. Let's take the communication skills we've learned and focus inward, because when we do, our health, performance, and our ability to enjoy our human experience can be taken to a whole new level.

In fall 2015, I volunteered at the Bulletproof Biohacking Conference in Pasadena, California. During this epic, three-day gathering of health-conscious consumers and cutting-edge health companies, I was grateful to be introduced to MyIntent Project, a jewelry company spreading love and intention through bracelets and necklaces. How does it work? If you are meeting with them in person as I was at the conference, they ask you a simple question: "What's your word?" What word describes what you're calling into your life right now? What one word gives voice to your intention at this point in your life?

After you tell them, they make a badass bracelet or necklace for you on the spot. Alternatively, you can order from their website (https://MyIntent.org) where you also have the option to use their "give back" feature to donate to the communities and countries from which they source the raw material used to make their jewelry.

Back in 2015, I didn't know exactly what I wanted to do or how to make it happen. I wasn't *clear*. I was all in my head and not in my heart. I wanted to be creative, but I wasn't sure how. I had all these stories coming up for me in my mind and I didn't feel at peace. I decided to follow the Four Levels of Truth-Telling discussed in chapter 3. I took a deep breath, tapped into my heart, and told the truth to myself. I tapped into my desire so I could operate from my truth—my highest calling—and actually *ask* for what I wanted.

So what was my one word?

Well, if you know me, you know I'm not one to always follow the rules. I think some rules are meant to be bent just a bit. So I asked for a bracelet with two words: "Create Clarity."

I was at a point in my life where I had so many ideas and interests, but didn't know how to channel them. I was living in Des Moines, Iowa, where I working for Clinical Health Coach. I was also writing this book. On top of these commitments, I had a strong calling to be creative in other areas of my life. I had a yearning for adventure, like living (or at least spending more time) in California, and going on a road trip from city to city to spread health to different communities.

What happened next? I asked for what I wanted from my boss—to work mobile office, spend more time in California, and travel the country spreading health from community to community. And after several months of wearing that bracelet, I'm excited to share that's exactly what happened. It wasn't easy. But with guidance, mentorship, and prayers, I took action on what I felt called to do.

This bracelet has served as a powerful reminder for me to create clarity about where I want to go and what I want to do with my life. It also led me to analyze my entire experience of creating clarity, and to really deconstruct the behind-the-scenes nuances of this process. I found there were a few steps that were absolutely key for me, and realized that others could benefit from the same joy, happiness, light, love, and health that comes from creating clarity—peace and health on earth. I call this concept The Circle of Clarity.

The Circle of Clarity:
Communicate→Relate→Think→Feel→Heal

There are five key concepts placed around The Circle of Clarity (see figure 2), forming a pentagram, that together can help us to create a new level of clarity in our lives.

The better we **communicate** with ourselves and others, the better we **relate** to everything and everyone (including ourselves) in our life. The better we relate to ourselves and others, the better we can **think** and **feel**. And finally, the better we can think and feel, the better we can **heal**.

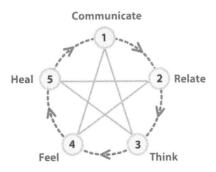

Figure 2. The Circle of Clarity.

1. Communicate

How we communicate with ourselves and others impacts how we relate. It all starts with communication. Not just through spoken words, but non-verbal communication as well. Our self-talk, thought patterns, body language, and written words all play a role in this concept of communication. If we can improve how we communicate with ourselves and others, we can improve how we relate to ourselves and others. The more clarity we can create in our communication, the more clarity and understanding we can create in our relationships.

2. Relate

We exist in relation to **everything** in this world. The key is possessing a conscious awareness of our most important relationships, those with ourselves, others, our planet, and our God. How we relate to these entities impacts how well we are able to function in our life.

3. Think

Remember, we are not our thoughts. But through our intention and action, we can influence our thoughts to help serve us in different areas of our lives.

4. Feel

How we think impacts how we feel (and vice versa). When we make the connection between how our thoughts and feelings interact with and affect each other, we soon realize that our thoughts can play tricks on us. And if our goal is to improve how we feel, we must look at how we think and all the areas of our life that impact (and are impacted by) how we think.

5. Heal

How we feel impacts how we heal—in the moment and in any stage of our lives. If there's some sort of physical ailment or sensation of stress being expressed, our ability to work and heal through this experience is crucial to our ability to grow and evolve in a healthy way. There is no shame in needing to heal. It can be quite freeing on a mental, physical, and emotional level. And when you do this, focus on your feelings—physically, in your body, and emotionally, in your heart. The phrase, "real healing comes from feeling" comes to mind. I believe feeling our feelings are foundational to any productive healing and behavior change process.

And now, if we tap into this intention of creating clarity, we can glide through life with ease and light, and with less stress and more happiness, in the direction of our dreams and our highest calling. If that's not a recipe for health, I don't know what is!

In my experience, healthy decision-making comes from the integration of feeling and thinking, allowing our minds to ask our bodies and hearts how they are and what they require. This multidimensional way of communicating starts with the breath in the present moment. The problem is most people are operating and making unconscious decisions without checking in with their bodies.

We need to evolve our decisions-making skills beyond the mind. When I make decisions, I try to ask myself what my body requires, not what my mind wants. And that starts with the breath.

Sometimes feelings can be a bit scary. Fear creeps in when we start to feel vulnerable. The mind is there to protect us. So when we have any type of fear— rational or irrational—the mind and the body go into protection mode. This event translates to suppressed emotions, mental resistance, limiting beliefs, increased cortisol (stress hormone) levels, and a lack of full, authentic feeling of what we're experiencing in the moment.

How can we deepen our capacity to feel? How can we go about feeling and then possibly share what we feel? One place to start is our approach to feelings in general.

Getting Better at Feeling

Have you ever read a book that changed the game for you? I mean literally created a reality shift, changing your perspective on life and the human experience up to this point?

That's what happened when I first read *The Presence Process* by Michael Brown. In my personal experience, this book provides the most powerful path to present moment awareness I've experienced. Hands down, one of the top ten books I've ever read. In his book, Brown explains that they goal is not just to feel better, but to get better at feeling. I also believe our capacity to reach optimal health and feel truly amazing is limitless, but our progress is stalled when we focus on trying to feel better and lose sight of the importance of getting better at feeling. We have the capacity not to control our feelings, but to mindfully listen and respond to them in an intentional and artful way.

Choose Presence

The Presence Process book is organized as a ten-week plan involving a new mantra to focus on each week. A core concept of this book is fostering consciously connected breathing. There are two, fifteen-minute breathing sessions suggested every day for ten weeks. Sounds like a lot, right?! I hear you. It's not *easy*, but it is simple.

I still use one of the main mantras from *The Presence Process* in my day to day life:

I. AM.   HERE. NOW.   IN. THIS.

And this is how you integrate it with your breath:

I. (INHALE)   AM. (EXHALE)

HERE. (INHALE) NOW. (EXHALE)

IN. (INHALE)   THIS. (EXHALE)

"What does *this* refer to?" you may be wondering. *This* is the present moment and each and every new present moment. There's a reason one of the 5 Ps of Health Hacking (from chapter 5) is Presence. If I were to rank these 5 Ps,

Presence would be number one. Presence is what will make or break someone's ability to reach the highest level of peace, love, health, and overall happiness.

I share this with you because these breathing sessions, and *The Presence Process* book in general, has made a profound impact on my life. It has helped me create clarity in all sorts of areas of my life and is a key process I use with health coaching clients. Maybe you've experimented with mantras and breathwork as well. Maybe you haven't. Either way, I've realized that if someone wants to feel better and truly get *real* with how they *feel* they may want to develop the willingness and interest to experiment with these types of practices. It may just be one of my favorite health hacks out there.

The secret to a balanced being is consciously connected deep breathing.

I believe we've hardly scratched the surface of what's possible with our capacity to fully *feel* our feelings. It may sound super cliché, but it's true. I believe, over time, we've been conditioned to suppress and not fully experience (let alone express), our emotions. In other words, it's not just about our capacity to feel, but how we process and integrate our feelings throughout our entire being. And when we are able to do this, we can watch our thoughts and behaviors unfold effortlessly throughout our day. We can accept this invitation to breathe, to feel, and to live in the present moment so we can communicate and relate to ourselves and everyone else with unconditional love and acceptance.

Summary:

- The Circle of Clarity is a simple concept to remind us of the connection between how we communicate, relate, think, feel, and heal.
- The first essential step to well-being and healing lies in our ability to truly experience our feelings.
- Many people focus on trying to feel better. This creates resistance to, rather than acceptance of, our current state. Instead, try focusing on the process of feeling—how you can get better at feeling.

Action Items:

1. What came up for you in this chapter? Can you relate to feeling overwhelmed and wanting clarity in your life now or in the past?

2. How can you put the Circle of Clarity into practice in your health and relationships?

3. What's your word? Do you have one or two words that speak to the intention your mind, body, heart, and soul are calling into your life? Consider choosing a word or two and ordering a necklace or bracelet from MyIntent Project at https://MyIntent.org. You can literally wear your intention on your body as a reminder of what you're calling into your life.

4. Feel Your Heart: Place your hand over your heart and feel your heartbeat. Notice your breath. Are you consciously breathing in a deep, connected way? If not, how can you add a little bit more conscious breathing into the moment?

5. **BONUS:** If you haven't already, consider reading *The Presence Process* by Michael Brown so you can experiment with the journey it provides.

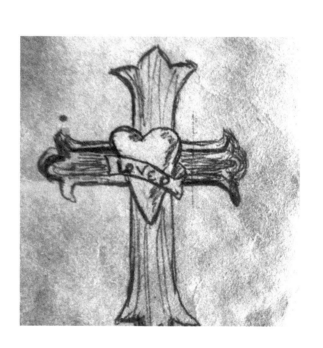

CHAPTER 8

You're Not Alone:

The Power of God and Close Relationships

*You are a creature of divine love connected at all times
to Source. Divine Love is when you see God in everyone
and everything you encounter.*
– WAYNE DYER

I'll be honest. This section took a lot of courage for me to write. But when I felt the fear, I knew it was an opportunity for growth.

Often times talking about God and spirituality does not come easy in our world. And I'm willing to bet when you first picked up this book about health hacking, you didn't think there would be a focus on spirituality. Think again.

I felt called to include the topics of God and spirituality because I'm writing this book from a place of my personal experience.

I'm not afraid to admit:

My faith and spiritual evolution have made a major impact on every area of my life and health.

My relationship with God and all divine energy has brought a lot of love, healing, peace, and power to my life. These relationships have allowed my ego to fade away and have helped me to realize there is more to explore outside of this human experience.

I grew up with a strong relationship with God and Jesus through the Catholic Church. I traveled to Italy, visited some of the most beautiful churches on earth, and eventually sang for the Pope in the middle of St. Peter's Square in Rome with my high school choir. And since then, I've learned about and grown to respect other ways of looking at religions, faith, and spirituality in general. These changes in my spiritual view have brought a lot of peace and deepening of relationships for me.

I won't try to sell you on believing in God or having a spiritual life. We are all on our own journey. I'm merely sharing what I've learned, what I've experienced, and how my relationship with God has impacted the quality of my entire life experience. Sharing these experiences through authentic self-expression brings me a lot of peace, and perhaps it will do the same for you. So here we go.

In my experience, multiple relationships support our personal quest for spiritual realization: our relationships with other humans and our relationships with God and the divine.

We grow and evolve in our spirituality by reading about those who came before us and by learning from those we interact with in the present moment. Furthermore, when we invite Spirit into our relationships, we invite the presence and love of God and the divine. Whether in person, over the telephone, or through written words, connecting with others in this way to gain different perspectives about life can yield beautiful realizations and new ways of loving and honoring ourselves and others. And this is why, if you recall from chapter 2, I chose to include Spirituality as one of the Four Areas of Macro Health. In each and every moment, we consciously (or subconsciously) choose to make decisions that impact our health, and deciding to incorporate spirituality in our lives is one of those choices.

Spirit on a Human Journey

While writing this book, I continued my own spiritual self-exploration by learning more about a philosophy known as Integral Theory. Integral Theory was created by Ken Wilber, author of several books, the first being *The Spectrum of*

Consciousness. In the foreword of his biography, *Ken Wilber: Thought as Passion*, Wilber defines the word "integral" and gives meaning to Integral Theory:

> The word *integral* means comprehensive, inclusive, non-marginalizing, embracing. Integral approaches to any field attempt to be exactly that—they include as many perspectives, styles, and methodologies as possible within a coherent view of the topic. In a certain sense, integral approaches are "meta-paradigms," or ways to draw together an already existing number of separate paradigms into a network of interrelated, mutually enriching approaches.

In my path of exploring integral theory and my quest to grow closer to God, I also stumbled upon a book called *Integral Christianity: The Spirit's Call to Evolve*. In this book, author Paul Smith presents an invitation to an "expansive pathway for the Christian religion that is faithful to a Jesus-centered theology of biblical interpretation and illuminated by the emerging field of integral philosophy."

"For most of my life I have believed that I was a human being on a spiritual journey," Smith notes in his book. "Now I believe that I am a spiritual being on a human journey." This shift in how we view our lives is quite interesting and empowering, depending on how you look at it. The more we can embrace our own spirituality, the closer we can grow to God.

Smith explains that whatever our religion is, most spiritual paths have many similarities, including the idea that spiritual practice for most people centers around prayer. Like Smith, I believe Christian, Buddhist, Jewish, Hindu—you name it—religions all share similar principles of prayer, meditation, and deep reflection.

Furthermore, Smith suggests that Jesus continues to be a prototype for all spiritual paths, and that, first and foremost, Jesus was a mystic:

> Mystical experience is available to everyone. It is a natural, normal part of our humanity until religion and society drive it out. Mystics are the normal people. It's the non-mystics who are abnormal!

For the mystic, God is present in nature, friendship, love, art, music, dance, laughter, suffering, pain, the poor, and the oppressed. We all have the potential to be modern-day mystics. It is already there deep inside us.

A Christian mystic is someone who most likely got to the mystical by looking at the life and teaching of Jesus. Others look at Buddha, or Krishna, or, as we all end up, looking inside. The mystics ask you to take nothing on mere belief. Rather, they give you a set of experiments to test within your own awareness and experience. The laboratory is your own mind and heart, the experiment is prayer and meditation, or whatever connects you to the Spirit.

This is my favorite part of his book as it shows us how we don't have to believe in God just for the sake of believing in God. We can actually experiment and test our experience of connecting with God. We can use our hearts and our minds to experiment with higher-state experiences to see what it might be like to connect with the Spirit.

Connecting with God Through Prayer

Have you ever experimented with your connection to and relationship with God?

As we consider different ways of doing this, let's start with prayer. Prayer doesn't have to be black or white. It can be a dynamic experience, full of color and vibrancy, that inspires a new, uplifting way of relating to God.

In his book, Smith presents **two types of prayer**:

- **Connecting Prayer.** We relate to spiritual realities in the world through thoughts, images, and ideas. We may have visualizations and hear messages from the Spirit.
- **Being Prayer.** We move away from dualism of relationship to Spirit into the unity of consciousness that Jesus had—oneness with God. In Being Prayer, we experience ourselves as Jesus experienced himself: as an infinite, divine being.

"Connecting Prayer" Story

During a different community gathering with friends, I experienced a special type of connecting prayer. I was surrounded by a few friends who were holding space for me as I shared about my struggle with spending time around people who didn't believe in God.

With my eyes closed, I had three images appear over the course of about two minutes. I saw Jesus' face, a cross, and a microphone. This was one of the more profound experiences I've had in connecting prayer. I felt that those images were symbols from God, calling me to trust in Jesus (Jesus' face), continue believing what I believe (the cross), and share what I believe with my voice (microphone). It was a deep healing experience to feel God calling to me in that moment.

Have you ever experienced anything similar to this type of connecting prayer?

We are divine infinite beings. Both connecting prayers and being prayers have a place in our world today. And so do the conversations about them.

Communicating with Feeling and Empathy

One of the great life lessons I've learned is to develop the capacity to communicate from a place of feeling.

Let's say you *want* to share something with someone but some fear comes up. You have ideas of what you *want* for yourself, but don't know how to go after them. Have you been there before? There is no clear blueprint to follow when sharing our feelings. But after we do the deep internal work of fully feeling our feelings, forgiving ourselves, telling ourselves the truth, or going through something like *The Presence Process* book, the next opportunity we have is to communicate and share with others

The Practice of "Circling"

About a year ago I first experimented with a way of communicating called "Circling." Developed by Integral Institute in Boulder, Colorado, Circling (also known as T3-Train the Trainer) is a creative and expansive practice designed to take our relationships to another level.

Circling is typically led by one person who moderates the exchanges between a small group of people. (In my experience, it works best when you have anywhere from two to five people present and involved.) This group of people sits in a circle and the moderator invites any one of the participants to volunteer to go first—to be the one "circled." This person shares something that they're currently thinking or feeling in that moment, or going through in their life. Then the other person (or the rest of the group) is invited to share what came up for them—what they *felt*, not thought—after hearing what that person shared.

This entire practice revolves around communicating from a place of feeling, and represents some of the most transformative conversations of which I've been a part. I've never felt so heard, appreciated, and understood for who I am. Imagine minimal feelings of judgment and maximum feelings of acceptance. It's pretty rad.

Why can't we do this health game on our own? Because we were meant to connect with other people. Why? To help each other heal, grow, and feel the freedom that comes from unconditional love and acceptance. Now if that's not a path toward human evolution, I don't know what is.

We're not alone, my friends. This form of self-expression allows us to be understood, not just by others, but by ourselves, in the most loving and accepting way possible. It helps us to process what we're feeling and thinking, who and what we are right now, and who and what we are becoming.

In my experience, the goal of spiritual growth isn't to get somewhere else, but to gradually wake-up to where we already are.

The techniques and skills needed to simultaneously grow in relationship with God and with others help us to wake up to the beauty of our current experiences.

No matter what you're feeling, no matter what you believe, and no matter your current relationships with the most important people in your life (and with God), I invite to understand and experiment with what else is possible.

By reading books that challenge or complement our current ways of thinking, and through heart-centered conversations with others, we can discover new, beautiful ways of relating to our families, friends, God, and everyone in between.

I believe God is everywhere. May we open our eyes, ears, hearts, and minds to witness God's divine love in everything and everyone around us.

Summary:

- Two Types of Prayer: Connecting Prayer and Being Prayer
- "Circling" is the practice of communicating from a place of feeling among a group of people in a way that takes relationships to another level. To learn more about the power of circling, visit IntegralCenter.org.
- Consider the idea that the purpose of spiritual growth isn't to get somewhere we are not currently at, but gradually wake up to where we already are.

Action Items:

1. How can you personally grow in relationship with God or the divine? How can you grow in relationship with others?
2. Do you read books about God or the divine? What have you learned from those books? Have you shared what you've learned with others?
3. If you go to church, do you do so out of habit or for some other reason?
4. Do you pray? If so, does prayer affect your mental and emotional state?
5. How do you communicate with others? Is it all in the head? Or with the heart?
6. **BONUS:** Choose God over gadgets. Take some time out of your schedule to pray and give thanks to God, Mother Earth, and all the divine. I challenge you to check your gadgets at the door, go outside, and enjoy peace and connection with your spiritual side.

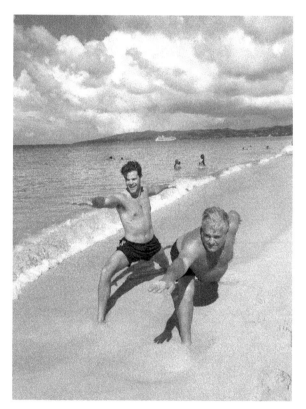

With my father, Scott, in St. Croix, U.S. Virgin Islands.

CHAPTER 9

Define Your Why:

Your Motive Means Everything

When you change the way you look at the things,
the things you look at change.
– Wayne Dyer

I'm willing to bet you probably thought we would be setting nutrition and workout goals for how to lose weight or get the perfect body by this point in the book. Don't worry. Setting those goals will come in the next few chapters, but first, let's talk about something equally important.

The last step in the Inner Game of Health starts with your *why*. Let's talk about understanding your motive, your purpose, and your reason for wanting the things what you want—peace, health, and vibrant energy, to name a few.

Our Health Blueprint

In the summer of 2014, I was on a plane flying back to Iowa from California reading a book called *Secrets of the Millionaire Mind*. In this book, author T. Harv Ecker describes the importance of getting clear on our *purpose* for wanting to build a millionaire mindset and achieve financial success. According to Ecker, "The roots create the fruit…If your motivation for acquiring money or success comes from a non-supportive root such as fear, anger, or the need to 'prove' yourself, your money will never bring you happiness."

Ecker goes on to describe how we all have a financial blueprint conditioned in our mind that's passed down from our parents, and that past programming and conditioning about money influences our relationship with money today. When I read this passage, the feelings that came up for me had *nothing* to do with money. When I read these words, it was like God threw a fastball, as fast as the ones my dad used to throw during batting practice as a kid, to my heart.

That's when I lost it. The emotions rolled in from my heart to my mind and permeated my entire body, ending in a lot of healing tears. You see, I realized that Ecker's message could be applied to our health—letting go of anger or resentment from the past. My father, whose stress from my parents' business sometimes affects his health, was one of my motivations and inspirations for learning more about health. I used to judge him for having this work-related stress. But after reading about how the roots create the fruit, I realized he was truly my hero. How he has cared for our family, built a business, and put all of us BEFORE HIMSELF—*that's* why he doesn't always live the healthiest life. He's focused on work so he can take care of our family. Can you relate?

When I returned home from my trip, instead of being angry at my father about his stress and for not eating healthy, I apologized for previously judging him. And I made sure I treated him and myself with love and compassion during the process.

When my interest in "improving" my health began, I was so focused on the *what* and the *how.* What would I need to do in order to achieve the outcomes I desired? What habits would I need to create? What behaviors would I need to change? And how would I do it?

Now, after some reflection, I've realized that adding the *why* behind all of these health changes has made the biggest impact.

Understanding your roots and defining your *why* for wanting to change your overall health can yield tremendous long-term results.

I've seen this happen first-hand with my clients. When people set goals they actually *want* to accomplish, a lot of progress can be made. Goal-setting can be powerful, but unless we define our *reason* for accomplishing the goal, it can easily go out the window. Or perhaps worse, we can achieve a goal through a process that lacks true meaning and purpose, resulting in an achievement that feels a bit worthless.

Remember, we all have a health blueprint that we are conditioned and programmed to live out from our childhood and passed down from previous generations. The key is to cultivate an awareness of this programming, as well as our roots and our motives, so we can integrate and transcend these realities in an intentional and loving way.

Intention Meets Attention

One of the most powerful concepts Michael Brown writes about in *The Presence Process* is understanding the value and opportunity that can be created when we allow our *intention* to meet our *attention*. This is another way of aligning our goals with our reasons for wanting to accomplish those goals.

Intention is the *why* of our focus, and our attention is the *what* of our focus. An intention can be anything we are hoping to achieve, and our attention is how we are going to make that thing happen. Here are some examples:

- If our intention is to foster closer relationships, we might focus our attention on making more eye contact in conversations.
- If our intention is to feel more rested in the morning, we might focus our attention on setting a bedtime and sticking to it.
- If our intention is to live a long, more energized life, we might focus our attention on scheduling a workout three times a week.
- If our intention is to eat more whole foods at home at eat fewer meals out, we might focus our attention on scheduling time to shop and prepare a healthy meal.

It doesn't matter what *it* is. We all have plenty of *its* in our lives. What's important is that the intention comes from the intersection of the heart, mind, body, and spirit. What if we were to take a step back and look at the bigger picture by asking ourselves a few questions to change the way we look at things?

Why now?

What questions can we ask ourselves and each other to allow our attention and intention to meet in support of our health journeys?

Here are a few:

- What's your intention?
- What's your reason why?
- Why is this important to you *right now*?
- Why are your health, energy, and performance important to you at *this particular moment* in your life?

Getting clear on the answers to these questions can create a cascade of connection between the heart, mind, body, and spirit, opening a door to your highest health and your best self.

Summary:

- We *all* have a health blueprints established in our childhood and passed down from previous generations. The key is creating clarity and having awareness around this and integrating it into our new health blueprints in an intentional and loving way.
- Defining our *why* is not just an important step in our quest for health improvement. It's integral. It's foundational. Without it, we lose sight of the reason why we are choosing to do what we are doing.

Action Items:

1. How has your health blueprint from childhood as well as your relationships with family members impacted your life? Are there specific areas of past programming about which you want to create, or have already created, more clarity?
2. Define Your *Why*. Why is your health important to you? If you want to make changes in your health, why is that important to you?

- This exercise is designed to help you set a foundation of why your health is important to you. Without this step, people tend to lose sight of the reason for making lifestyle changes. They also lose focus and success rates fall dramatically.
- **Friendly tip:** Do this exercise in a comfortable place—a place you really love. This could be your favorite coffee shop, your office, your couch, or your tree house. Just find a place where you can relax and spend some time thinking about these questions.

ACT 4

Getting Started:

Take Inventory and Take Action!

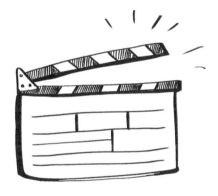

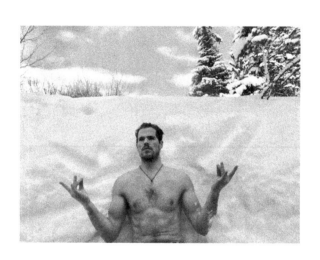

CHAPTER 10

Take a Break, Take a Breath:

How to Assess and Express This Thing We Call Stress

In times of stress, the best thing we can do for each other is to listen with our ears and our hearts and to be assured that our questions are just as important as our answers.
– MISTER ROGERS

The time has come to acknowledge the work you've done up to this point. Most people miss out on the ground work—the inner game of health we have explored so far. Instead, they usually go straight into action mode. Not you, my friend.

We've covered some higher-level health topics as well as deep emotional and spiritual topics. I shared some personal stories to give you a glimpse into how I've grown and what I've learned about managing my own emotions. But before we start mapping a plan of action to change some behaviors in our health, it's important we take inventory of and reflect on one of the more important areas of our health—our relationship with *stress*.

In a world where it's easy to get caught up in the patterns and routines of life, slowing down to assess our stress is quickly becoming a lost art.

According to the American Psychology Association's (APA) 2010 Stress in America survey, 44 percent of adults in the United States report their level of stress has increased in the last five years. Stress is also being studied for its effect on not only our short-term health and quality of life, but perhaps more importantly, the future of our existence. Multiple studies are linking stress with shorter telomeres, a chromosome component that's been associated with aging and increased risk of developing diabetes, heart disease, and cancer.

In this section, let's consider how (and when) stress shows up in our lives; the difference between real, remembered, and imagined stress; as well as a few practices to consider experimenting with in our daily and weekly routines to support our ability to have a healthy relationship with stress. Remember, if the goal is to change patterns of dis-ease in our life, we must embrace new ways of doing things rooted in health-ease.

When I work with some coaching clients who are hungry for a health upgrade or an overall boost in energy and performance, they often want to rush the actions. They know where they want to be and they want to get there as fast as possible. This might work for some, especially if they're in action mode. But if you are someone who wants to ease into the action, go right ahead. In fact, it's highly encouraged. By easing into the action phase of behavior change, we stay focused on the present. Remember, we can't change time, we can only change our relationship to it.

Whether in your mind or in your daily habits, I'm willing to bet you are currently experimenting with a new habit or behavior.

Am I correct?

So let me ask, what steps (in your mind, your heart, or your actions) did you take to prepare for this new habit?

Did you assess your stress?

Taking a moment to reflect on and assess your stress in this moment and in this stage of your life (before you move forward with a full-on health action plan), can yield so many benefits.

Why? Because if we're already stressed out, adding nutrition changes or workout plans will build more stress on top of stress.

Don't lose the beautiful art of self-reflection in our everyday lives, especially when you plan for and begin to take action.

Stress and Technology

In a 2017 survey, the APA found almost two-thirds (65 percent) of Americans somewhat or strongly agree that periodically "unplugging" or taking a "digital detox" is important for their mental health. However, of those individuals, only 28 percent report following through with their interest in stepping away from technology. In the same survey, the APA also found those who constantly check email, texts, and social media report higher levels of stress.

Just the other day, I was talking with a lovely mother of two named Elizabeth. We discussed the topic of technology and the role smartphones play in our society. She shared about an article that discussed how we are starting to lose the art of self-reflection in our everyday lives.

She also pointed out that whenever we have a break from doing something that requires our attention, we tend to take that break with our phones.

Think about it for a moment.

Elizabeth was right. When we have a free moment, we go to straight to our phones. We check our emails, text messages, phone calls, calendar, and our favorite social media channels. Furthermore, when we are performing a particular action while multitasking on our phones (i.e., opening a door, driving a car), we're not fully present in that primary action or moment. For some, our phones are in our beds, our bathrooms, our kitchens, our offices, and everywhere we go in public.

These so-called "smart" devices are present in a majority of our moments, but how smart are they really making us?

The idea isn't to necessarily go cold turkey, ditching these devices in the street and running into the forest without any technology at all. Instead, begin by simply building awareness around your relationship with technology. Recognize that smartphones and social media are *not* essential to human life. And remain present in every moment. Technology can be a tool, but it requires intentional awareness and action to use it properly.

In the book *Alone Together: Why We Expect More from Technology and Less from Each Other*, Sherry Turkle makes the case for technology forming the basis of one's identity. "The self shaped in a world of rapid response measures success by calls made, emails answered, texts replied to, contacts reached. This self is calibrated on the basis of what technology proposes." She goes on to say that each of us has our own distinct online, virtual identity, which is mostly developed via our smartphone connectivity. Is she right? Depending on when you grew up, your identity has most likely been influenced in some way by your smartphone and social media.

The truth is simple, but hard for some people to deeply understand.

YOU ARE NOT YOUR FACEBOOK PROFILE.

YOU ARE NOT YOUR INSTAGRAM PAGE.

YOU ARE NOT YOUR SNAPCHAT.

Whatever technology or social media platforms you use for work or play, it's time to create some clarity and realize how they impact our identity and our way of life.

For the record, I used to use my smartphone for everything; however, in the past few years, I've become more aware of how often I use it when it isn't 100 percent necessary.

Let's continue to explore, arguably, the single greatest cause of poor health— our stress.

Assess Your Stress

According to Dr. Mark Hyman, the medical definition of stress is "the *perception* of a real or imagined threat to your body or your ego."

Stress is deeply affected by stories created in our minds, as dramatically impacted by the behaviors and habits that make up our lifestyle. Evolutionarily speaking, and in some emergency situations today, stress can be considered highly adaptive—stress brought on by a flight or fight reaction to a real or perceived threat in the environment ensured survival of an individual and the human species. But in today's world, we've developed a skewed reality of what *real* stress is. Most of us don't have as many truly stressful dangers as we may think. For example, if I'm late to a meeting, missing my phone charger, or trying to meet a deadline for work, it's easy for me to lose sight of my breath, allow my brain to take over, and fall into an intense stress-response mode in my body.

Can you relate?

But here's the thing—not all stress is bad.

For example, stress is required to produce training adaptations when exercising. In order to learn something with a moderate to high degree of focus and difficulty, you need to stress your brain in new ways. As humans we're designed to handle acute (or intermittent) amounts of stress, just not *chronic* amounts of stress.

Do you think you have any symptoms of chronic stress?

- Insomnia
- Low energy
- Mood swings
- Upset Stomach
- Loss of sexual desire
- Aches, pains, and tense muscles

Take a Break and Take a Breath

In this moment, take inventory of your current level of stress, and reflect on times in your life when you feel a bit more stressed.

- How stressed are you feeling now? Where do you feel your stress? How would you describe this stress?
- How do you usually handle stress in your life?
- Are there certain people, environments, or times of the day that bring about stress in your life?

- When was the last time you gave yourself a break?

Whether you choose to take a fifteen-minute work break to walk outside, or choose to give yourself an emotional break after something stressful occurred, we all deserve to make that choice. I've been there before, with family, work, money issues, or when something is not going my way. What usually helps me work through the moment is the conscious, intentional choice to give myself a break. And the choice usually starts with the breath.

Go ahead, take a break and breathe for a moment, checking in with how you are relating to stress in this moment and in your life in general.

Inhale deeply into the stomach and audibly exhale.

Just Breathe.

How does it feel?

Could you possibly use more intentional breathing in your life?

If so, keep reading. I have a fun exercise for you.

There are several hacks you can integrate into your lifestyle to support your body's stress response; however, there is only one that I find essential in my own life as a daily ritual. And that is mastering the breath.

Instead of asking ourselves questions like, what can I *do* to stress less, it's important to realize it's not the lack of *doing* that causes our stress. It's the lack of *being* in the moment with our breath. In my experience, integrating consciously connected breathing into the present moment is the first step toward preventing, releasing, and managing our stress.

If you think about it, being mindful of the breath requires some intention, but not that much difficult action. The breath is an interesting bodily function, as it is an autonomic (involuntary) aspect of our physiology, meaning it will happen no matter what, without our influence. However, we can also add conscious, thoughtful intention to influence our breath. The question is—how can we help ourselves remember to breathe deeply and intentionally?

The Feedback Loop of Presence

Based on my past experiences, I created a feedback loop to remind me of the intention I can add to my process of breathing. Breathing just for the sake of breathing can be quite helpful, but if we add some intention to our experience, it can also lead to new levels of feeling and awareness in our lives.

Note: The breath is involved in each step of this process and not just at the beginning. This is a practice you can use during any part of your day.

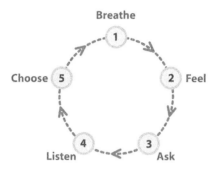

The Feedback Loop of Presence

1. Breathe

Breathe deep into your heart and your stomach. Let your lungs fill up and then let the air flow through your body and out of your mouth and nose.

2. Feel

Feel from a place of observation and non-judgment. As you start to feel more, you will begin to *feel better,* but again, as we learned from Michael Brown in chapter 7, it's not about feeling better, it's about getting better at feeling.

3. Ask

Ask yourself some open-ended questions: What am I noticing? How do I feel called to respond? What response would be in my best and highest interest?

4. Listen

Listen to your heart and body as you await the answers to your questions. And just notice the feelings.

5. Choose

Choose a response that's in alignment with your best and highest self, and return to the beginning of the feedback loop with the breath.

This feedback loop serves as a model for our minds to follow in our quest for creating peaceful presence in our lives. Here are a few more hacks and breathing exercises to follow in support our body's ability to manage our stress properly.

The Power of Breathwork

Integrating any sort of daily practice of breathwork for stress management can be a powerful habit with benefits that carry over into other areas of your life. It's not necessarily that every moment calls for these exact breathing techniques, but a majority of the moments we experience in this world have some level of stress involved. And having some sort of breathing practice under our belt can be very helpful. If you've practiced yoga, you're probably familiar with some breathing exercises already. Here are a few to try:

Exercise 1: Alternate Nostril/Yogic Breathing

This first example may be new for you, or it may already be a daily ritual you practice. Either way, it's important to consistently practice something as fundamental as breathing.

Take a deep, full, and relaxed breath as you follow the sequence below. It's important to heed the word "relaxed." We can easily take deep and full breaths in a quick, stressful way. But we're aiming to relax, so invite that intention into your breathing practice. Consider following this sequence for three to five minutes:

1. Inhale through the left nostril with your right nostril closed by your right thumb.

2. Exhale through your right nostril with your left nostril closed by your right index or ring finger.

3. Repeat.

It's simple enough to do, but requires just the right amount of focus to move the fingers back and forth and to adjust the pace of the breath.

Exercise 2: Wim Hof Method

If we want to settle our mind, body, or emotions in the world we live in today, we need to get a bit creative. I'm talking out-of-the-comfort-zone creative. And that's exactly what Wim Hof did when he designed his own (some call it revolutionary) breath practice.

Named after a middle-aged Dutchman, the Wim Hof Breathing Method has had a radical impact on my life by transforming how I breathe and how I influence my autonomous nervous system, resulting in next-level performance, feeling, clarity, and present-moment awareness. It has also taught me how to be more conscious of my breath throughout the day.

If you do a Google search of Wim Hof, you'll find some photos and videos of this radical health hacker and self-proclaimed "Iceman" sitting in the middle of a giant piece of ice, just chilling. (Pun intended.) He holds twenty Guinness World Records for withstanding extreme temperatures—he has stayed in ice baths for multiple hours, climbed Everest and Kilimanjaro in only shorts and shoes, and ran a marathon in 122°F heat with no water or food. Crazy, right?! Not to him. To him, it's a way of life that can radically transform the way we manage our health and immune system in the world today.

I had the honor of witnessing Hof's surprise visit to the 2015 Bulletproof Biohacking Conference. He was not expected to attend the conference, but made a surprise visit at the last minute to lead a room full of more than four hundred people through his powerful breath exercise. He brought the house down, so to speak. Not just for the amazing feeling and sensation that his method creates, but because of his awesome, happy-go-lucky personality. His energy just lights you up.

So what is his method, exactly?

The Wim Hof Method is based on three core pillars—cold therapy, breathing, and commitment (or mindset). Together, when done correctly, these three pillars can work wonders for boosting the immune system and feeling more powerful. At least they have for me.

For the purposes of this section, we will focus on the breathing pillar, which also involves the commitment or mindset pillar.

Here are the five steps of the Wim Hof breathing practice explained:

1. **Get comfortable.** Sit in a meditation posture or lie down flat with your back on the floor. Doing it first thing in the morning on an empty stomach is suggested, but you can do it later in the day too.

2. **Power breaths.** Once you're comfortable, you can start to slowly breathe in and out thirty times. Imagine you're blowing up a balloon and your body is being saturated with fresh oxygen; not too shallow and not too deep. Inhale through the nose and exhale through the mouth in short powerful bursts. Inhale, stomach fills up with oxygen. Exhale, stomach sinks in as you release the breath. This may feel a bit like you are hyperventilating, and this is normal (but you are in control, of course).

   Note: Watch your heart rate during this exercise. The heart rate may naturally rise, but it's important not to let it rise to the point that you lose comfort in the practice.

3. **Feel your body.** Notice what your body is feeling while you're engaging in this breathing exercise. Notice the sensations in your hands, arms, legs, lungs, face, and jaw. Notice where in your body you're holding on to stress and relax into that area. Imagine your energy moving throughout your body as you engage in these breaths.

4. **Hold and release.** After doing twenty to thirty rapid breaths over about thirty seconds, draw the breath in once more and fill the lungs to maximum capacity without using too much force. Then push all the air out and hold the breath for as long as you comfortably can. Relax and notice the energy channels in your body and how the oxygen is spreading around. If you'd like, this is when you can measure the length of your breath hold by setting a timer. You can also close your eyes

during this breath hold. And to take it to the next level, do some push-ups or yoga poses during this breath hold. (I've found I can hold my breath longer when my body changes positions or when I do push-ups.)

5. **Breathe in for ten to fifteen seconds.** After the breath retention, release that breath and take another deep breath in and hold it for another ten to fifteen seconds before exhaling.

Warning: It's important to note that you must follow these steps with careful intention. According to http://WimHofMethod.com, it's important to follow the practice the way it is explained and avoid practicing the method in the wrong environment. Here is an important message from their website:

The breathing exercise has a profound effect and should be practiced in the way it is explained. Always do the breathing exercise in a safe environment (e.g., sitting on a couch/floor) and unforced. Never practice the exercises before or during diving, driving, swimming, taking a bath or in any other environment/place where, should you pass out, a serious injury could occur. Wim Hof breathing may cause tingling sensations and/or lightheadedness. If you've fainted, it means that you went too far. Take a step back next time…Do not practice the method during pregnancy or when having epilepsy. Persons with cardiovascular health issues, or any other (serious) health conditions, should always consult a medical doctor before starting with the Wim Hof Method.

And there you have the Wim Hof Method.

Additional Stress Management and Recovery Hacks

In addition to breathing exercises, there are several other stress-minimizing hacks I love to follow. Here are five of my go-to strategies for creating a healthier relationship with stress:

1. Float Tanks

Float tanks, also called sensory deprivation tanks, are lightless, soundproof tanks where people float in a thousand pounds of salt water at skin temperature for hours at a time. The result? The body relaxes and the only sensation you experience is your breath, your digestive system, and your mind.

These sensory deprivation tanks were first created and used by National Institutes of Health researcher, physician, and neuroscientist, John C. Lilly, in 1954. The goal? To observe the effects of complete sensory deprivation and help people dial down the mind and sense of self.

Over the past decade, float tanks have gained popularity as a new tool for meditation and relaxation, as well as a treatment method in the field of alternative medicine. I'm an avid floater, going about once every month or so for the past few years. And in my experience, my ability to feel—in a deep and clear way— has become incredibly heightened. My jaw, my shoulders, my stomach, and, perhaps most importantly, my breath, have all relaxed in a very noticeable way. If you haven't tried float tanks yet, I'd recommend putting them toward the top of your list.

2. Self-Massage

Where do you carry your stress? For me, it's in my jaw, neck, and shoulders. One of my daily habits is to check in with my body and provide a little self-care by massaging myself with my own hands. This may seem too simple to be listed as a stress-management solution, but if used properly, self-massage can make a big impact on reducing stress levels.

To take it to the next level, you can invest in one of the following self-massage or myofascial release tools I've used in the past. As you can see, there is no shortage of options to consider:

- Trigger Point Foam Roller–A great standard foam roller, easy to travel with and intended for full-body roll out
- MyoBuddy Massager Pro–A high-powered, professional grade, vibrational device great for deep tissue massage and myofascial release
- Standard Lacrosse Balls–Great for travel and easy to use on feet or other areas of pain
- The Oh Ball Premium Massage Ball Roller—Great for plantar fasciitis or any other type of foot pain
- The Rolflex (i.e., the foam roller reimagined)–Easy to travel with, this innovative two-piece device allows for stabilized trigger point and active

release application unlike any other standard foam roller. The unique shape provides pressure without restricting motion and can be self-administered without rolling on the ground.

- The Balsaq–With the most fitting name possible, this mobility tool includes two lacrosse balls inside of a stretchy sack. I met the co-founder, Dr. Christy Verges, and tried out her invention at a health conferences, and was blown away. The design allows for a certain type of recovery and mobility you just can't get with one lacrosse ball.

- The Wave Tool–This is my new favorite tool. I was introduced to The Wave Tool by Laura, my physical therapist in Boulder, Colorado. She created the wave tool for practitioners, like massage therapists and physical therapists, to use with their patients. But it can also be used as a tool to treat yourself or your loved ones. It's a small and hard handheld tool with specific types of edges designed to be used for self-massage and also for soft tissue immobilization—to help break up scar tissue, promote blood flow, and ease chronic tendonitis and fascia (connective tissue) pain.

3. Light Movement and Grounding

One of the most underrated ways to lower stress is through light movement. Don't underestimate the power of a peaceful walk outside. Whenever I feel stressed by something in my work or personal life, I find taking a twenty-minute walk outside does wonders to relax my mind and awaken my senses. And if I have access to grass, I prefer to take my shoes off to soak up the negative ions from the soil of Mother Earth (referred to as "grounding").

4. Temperature Change

Cleaning ourselves in the shower is a key part of maintaining healthy hygiene. Depending on the temperature you choose, you can also support your body's stress response.

- Hot or warm showers and baths can relieve tension and soothe stiff muscles. They can also increase levels of the all-too-powerful "love hormone," oxytocin. If you have a powerful showerhead, you can let the hot water work like a mini-massage on your shoulders, neck, and back. Or if you decide to take a warm bath, you can add a few scoops of Epsom salts (magnesium sulfate), which have been found to support the recovery of sore muscles.

Note: Some believe magnesium chloride (a different form of magnesium) may even be more effective than Epsom salts (magnesium sulfate). You can usually find both at your local grocery store or online. A well-respected brand is EnviroMedica, but choose the one that's right for you.

- Cold showers or ice baths, as uncomfortable as they can seem, actually work wonders for our bodies. Turning the water to cold for the last few minutes of a shower can help wake the body and mind. This quick change in temperature relieves the body of fatigue and increases mental alertness. And if you have any sort of injury, an ice bath may also be helpful.

  Note: Cold water is actually better for our hair and skin; whereas a hot shower can dry us out, a cold shower hydrates our body.

5. Supplements and Drinks.

- **Cannabidiol (CBD)** is the non-psychoactive component found in marijuana. Completely legal in all fifty states, CBD is a great supplement used to relax the mind and body, as well as ease headaches or physical pains. I use CBD all the time. It's not cheap, but it's one of my favorite go-to supplements. CBD can also be great to spark creative thinking, without the unwanted side effects of "getting high" (from THC). I'm a big fan and ambassador of EAD Labs, the makers of BioCBD—arguably the best CBD on the market.

- **Chamomile** is an herb often consumed in tea form to help ease an upset stomach and relax you before bed. It is readily available at your local grocery store or online.

- **Kava (or Kava Kava)** is a root from the Pacific islands, where people have used it for centuries as a pain reliever. Kava is also great to help you manage anxiety—promoting relaxation, but allowing you to maintain focus as needed. Kava can most likely be found in a tea bag form at your local grocery or health food store.

- **Reishi Mushrooms** are known to be great for the nervous system and immune system, supporting a calm state in the body. My favorite brand is Four Sigmatic, as they source some of the cleanest mushrooms on the planet. They make on-the-go, individual-serving, travel packs. One option is Reishi by itself, and the other is Reishi with Hot Cacao. Check out the other mushrooms they sell as well, including Lions Mane (great for brain health, mental focus, and nervous system health), Cordyceps (great for physical energy and lung health), Chaga (excellent for the immune system), and even Mushroom Coffee (which will turn your brain on to a new level of focus and energy)!

You don't have to follow any of my favorite health hacks, the Feedback Loop of Presence, or different breathing methods right now or in the future. But you can still learn about these stress-minimizing habits and consider experimenting with them as a new practice in your life.

Above all, remember that whenever you're feeling a bit tired or stressed out, you can always take a break and take a breath.

Summary:

- Nearly two-thirds (65 percent) of Americans somewhat or strongly agree that periodically "unplugging" or taking a "digital detox" is important for their mental health; however, only 28 percent of those individuals report following through with their interest in stepping away from technology.
- Individuals who constantly check email, texts, and social media report higher levels of stress.
- Practice the Feedback Loop of Presence: Breathe, Feel, Ask, Listen, and Choose

- Learning to create a conscious practice of self-reflection in our daily lives is integral to fostering healthy relationships with anything from our smartphones and the present moment to ourselves and others.
- Using different breathing exercises, movements, temperature changes, and supplements can allow your body to lower its current level of stress and feel more at ease.

Action Items:

1. What is your relationship like with technology? Consider both the quantity and quality of your technology use. Do you need a higher or lower quantity, or just a better quality, of technology in your life?
2. During which part(s) of your day do you feel most stressed?
3. Try a new breathing exercise: Alternate Nostril/Yogic Breathing or the Wim Hof Breathing Method are two solid options.
4. What time of day might you want to try out these new practices? Whenever you get stressed or at a specific time of day (e.g., first thing in the morning, over a lunch break, or before bed) to help build them as a habit?

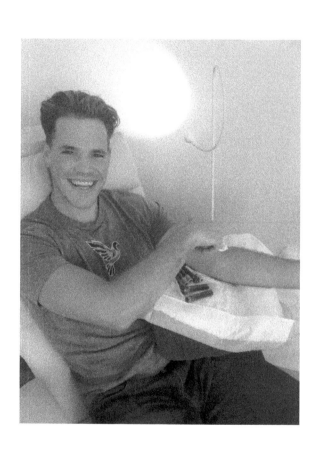

CHAPTER 11

Measure What Matters:

Advanced Blood Testing and Hacking Your Genetics

Not only are our genes powerful, but they are also malleable and programmable-they are never static...you must realize that your genes are not your destiny, but they are your tendency.
– ANDREW ROSTENBERG, D.C.

The human mind is hungry for improvement, but it also wants to avoid failure, danger, and, ultimately, death. As I shared earlier, my visit to the ER for dehydration may have seemed harmless; but the truth is, I may have been a cup or two of coffee away from extreme dehydration, and eventual death, due to low sodium levels.

Throughout this book, I've talked a lot about the emotional and spiritual side of health and human consciousness. If you desire to live a long, happy life with less stress and fewer sick days, more energy and focus, and an overall better quality of life, we must look beyond how we feel and our relationships to consider some important science.

We must work to make the connection between how we think and feel to how we are doing at the cellular level—in our blood and DNA—to truly understand our current and future state of health. Yes, sometimes nerding out on some science (or at least taking a small interest in learning) can be helpful in our quest for health optimization and positive behavior change.

Earlier, we talked a little bit about the Quantified Self movement. I don't know about you, but measuring every little thing in my life feels overwhelming. So instead of measuring everything, let's focus on the most important things.

In this chapter, we'll consider measuring some interesting (and important) biomarkers and dive into advancements in direct-to-consumer lab testing, including blood work, genetic testing, and other pieces of information like Heart Rate Variability (HRV). Measuring our daily steps, weight, and body fat percentage might give us a feeling of accomplishment, but if we want to optimize our health for the long haul, we'll need to think outside the box, or inside the body, rather, to measure other important areas of our health.

The information we gather from these tests can allow us to master prevention in our life.

But first, what is prevention? The term prevention is often overused and misused in our world today. Prevention is getting good sleep and sunlight, as well as consuming quality, local, whole foods. Prevention is moving our bodies, having fun with friends, and also knowing our blood work. In contrast, getting a mammogram or a colonoscopy every year beginning at a certain age is *not* prevention. It's early detection. While our doctor may tell us "everything looks good" after reading mammogram or blood work results, there are always opportunities for improvement with respect to prevention.

What do you measure to prevent disease and optimize health?

In chapter 4, I asked you to reflect on the main quantitative and qualitative information you track and measure in your health. Do you remember what you wrote? Go back and review what you shared.

In the current chapter, we will dive a bit deeper to help you compare what you *currently* measure with some of the most important things you *could* measure.

Do you own any wearable technology, such as a FitBit or an Oura Ring?

Do you step on the scale every day, or at least once a week, to measure your weight?

Do you track all of the weight you lift, including sets, reps, and other details of your workouts?

If so, good for you! That sort of commitment to your health can help you start measuring other health data that might be even more important in your quest for a long, peaceful, and healthy life.

If you don't measure any health information, that's ok too! Together we'll create some clarity about some of the important information you can begin to measure.

Again, I want to mention I am not a doctor or trained medical professional offering medical advice. I am a health coach and health hacker who has chosen to learn about different biomarkers in my health. Unfortunately, this quest came not from a specific interest in prevention, but out of necessity following my visit to the emergency room.

My Visit to the ER—The "Hacker" Emerges

In 2015, I started experimenting with a high fat, low carb, ketogenic diet. The goal? To burn fat easier, feel better, think clearer, and prevent illness.

The ketogenic diet is high in healthy fat, low in crappy carbs, and includes moderate amounts of protein, all aimed at helping change how your body burns fuel—shifting from using carbs or glucose for fuel, to using fat or ketones as fuel.

The ketogenic diet was originally made famous for its therapeutic role in helping patients with epilepsy in the 1920s and 1930s, but has gained a lot of popularity over the past decade for its diverse health benefits, including burning fat quicker and regulating blood sugar, as well as helping to prevent diabetes, cancer, and other diseases such as Alzheimer's. This way of eating can also get you into a state of ketosis, where the brain and body are literally running off of a different fuel source—ketones instead of glucose. But it can also lead to dehydration and cause your blood work to change pretty quickly.

While eating this way, it seemed easier to burn fat, I felt like I had more energy, and I felt like I had more mental clarity overall. But I also started to notice how sensitive my body was to caffeine. Fast-forward to early 2016, and the ketogenic diet combined with too much caffeine and not enough sodium landed me in the hospital for dehydration.

I'll never forget it. I was in the middle of brunch with my family on a Sunday afternoon when I started to feel "off." You know, that feeling of being light-headed and feeling itchy on my head. I had a few coffees and a green tea at brunch. And I wasn't feeling too hot.

I went to the bathroom to see if splashing some water on my face would help. Not so much. On my way back to the table, I slowly went from walking to down on my knees. That's when I started going in and out of consciousness. The next thing I knew, I was in a booth at the restaurant after my sister had jammed an epinephrine auto-injector into my leg (she thought I may be having an allergic reaction to something I'd eaten). Before the day was done, I had received two epi-pen (epinephrine) shots, one in each leg, a shot of Benadryl, and a nice mix of fluids in the ER after an ambulance ride to the hospital.

Practicing what I preach in my health is very important to me, but I'll admit, I'm not perfect. And I wasn't perfect in my health on this day and the days leading up to my visit to the ER.

Now, I know what you may be thinking. How could someone who is so "healthy" have such a crazy health scare? Well, you know the ketogenic diet I had been on? That, combined with a few other factors, sent my minerals out of whack. According to conversations with my naturopathic doctor and friends, I was extremely dehydrated with deathly low sodium levels.

Here are a few things I believe contributed to my visit to the ER:

- In going to a ketogenic diet, I cut out some hydrating foods, including fruits and some other veggies. I was not eating enough vegetables and not properly making up for my loss in minerals.
- I was not properly hydrating around my workouts. Plus I was pushing it a bit in my workouts. I wanted to avoid bad sources of sugar and had not found alternative sources to use for hydration.
- I was not eating enough salt on my foods, especially early in the day. Which is interesting, because this was one of the first hacks I learned about while doing research for this book—it's very important to

consume a pinch or two of high quality sea salt upon waking up as it can help your adrenals use energy better.

- And last, but certainly not least, I had consumed too much caffeine—both that morning and the days and weeks leading up to it—which can dehydrate you by directly lowering sodium levels.

I learned a lot that day. Not the least of which is that caffeine is a drug. It is not essential. Does coffee have healthy components to it? Yes. Can we use it as a tool to help us improve our mental performance? Yes. However, I now vote for decaf over caffeine any day of the week, especially for people who are sensitive to caffeine and don't get enough high-quality salt. And I caution people to realize too much caffeine can cause a lot more harm than good. Through this experience, I also learned the value of measuring my blood work as I make lifestyle changes as drastic as I did.

My ER experience actually happened as I was in the middle of writing this book. And I'm grateful it did, because it has led me down a path of continued learning about how I can measure what matters in my body and act accordingly.

So how can we get started measuring what matters?

The way I see it, there are two different types of data involved: Performance and Fitness Tracking data, and Essential Health Tracking data (with some overlap between these two categories):

- **Performance/Fitness Tracking data** (e.g., measuring steps, calories burned, ketone levels, number of workouts in a week, time spent outdoors in the sun, etc.)
- **Essential Health Tracking data** (e.g., genetic data, full-scale blood work, body fat/composition, micronutrient deficiency levels, heart-rate variability, heavy metal testing, microbiome or gut health testing, etc.)

For the purposes of this chapter, we will focus on the following categories of Essential Health Tracking data:

1. Know Your Blood Work

2. Know Your Genetics
3. Know Your Nutrients
4. Know Your Stress (through HRV)

I have highlighted these four principles to follow when hacking and tracking your most important health markers, as well as companies I recommend to assist you in this process. I will also share what I've learned in the process of doing my own Essential Health Tracking and how you can follow suit. Enjoy!

Principle 1: Know Your Blood Work

Having needles stuck in my veins is not my idea of fun. So when I decided I would start hacking my blood work two years ago, I realized I'd have to reframe how I viewed this procedure. I needed to increase my level of perceived importance of the test and my level of confidence that I would survive. Furthermore, I believed that taking this intentional action would, in fact, help me thrive by allowing me to learn more about what was going on inside my body.

To give you some context, in early 2015, I was about six months into experimenting with a ketogenic-esque (high fat, low carb, moderate protein) diet. We're talking about 70 to 80 percent of calories from fat. I had been doing a self-study on the topic of ketogenic diets, and specifically the true causes of heart disease. One of the books I read was *Cholesterol Clarity: What the HDL is Wrong with My Numbers* by Jimmy Moore and Dr. Eric Westman. In this book, Moore and Westman present interviews with leading experts on the topic of heart health, cholesterol, and saturated fat. I learned a lot about heart health, including how our society's widespread fear of eating fat in food is largely mistaken. Additionally, I learned about the politics involved with Big Pharma and how they play a role in creating the cholesterol reference ranges our standard clinics use today, leading to an overconsumption of statin drugs.

It is often said annual blood work is the most important thing adults can do to stay on top of their health. And in general, I agree. But that doesn't mean you have to simply go to your doctor for an annual screening and they tell you you're fine or suggest that you eat less of this or that. I believe we're called to play more of an active role in our health *beyond* annual visits. That includes understanding the most important lab work to have done and asking our health care team about these tests.

Nowadays, most people simply depend on doctors to tell them when something is going wrong in their health. But the consumers who want to play more of an active role in their health can also bring questions and ideas directly to their doctor.

In reality, many physicians lack both the time and resources to provide a complete overview of your biomarkers. There is a growing movement known as direct-to-consumer lab testing, with dozens of companies providing opportunities for consumers to test their own biomarkers without standing in long lines, and for some, not even leaving home. Talk about a revolutionary approach to health care.

How does it work?

As an example, WellnessFX is a company that offers different blood testing kits for consumers to purchase online. A consumer then schedules an appointment directly with WellnessFX's partner lab, Quest Diagnostics, one of the most well-known and respected labs in the US.

The first test I purchased was the "Advanced Heart Health" test. Using ion mobility fractionation, this test goes beyond most traditional lipid panel tests to understand what's really going on inside your heart.

What is ion mobility fractionation and why is this type of testing important to you?

Ion mobility fractionation is the latest technology in the evolution of advanced lipid subclass measurements, going beyond the standard means of measuring Total Cholesterol, Total HDL, and Total LDL. This process breaks down lipoproteins on the basis of size and concentration, measuring small, medium, and total LDL particle numbers. For a glimpse of my lab work hosted on WellnessFX's secure online portal, see figure 3 and figure 4.

Figure 3 shows my basic lipid panel—Total Cholesterol, HDL, LDL, and Triglycerides. Figure 4 shows a breakdown of my LDL particles and HDL particles, two areas of heart health not traditionally measured by standard tests. Green indicates levels in the optimal range, orange indicates moderate levels, and red indicates higher risk. As you can see, the majority of my levels are in the green category; however, I do have a few levels in the orange and red. This means there is room for improvement.

(I have been supplementing on and off with niacin, cycling on and off a keto diet, and have made some other smaller tweaks to my diet and lifestyle that are affecting my levels. My hypothesis is that my body is getting used to a high fat diet, and the levels will most likely normalize over time.)

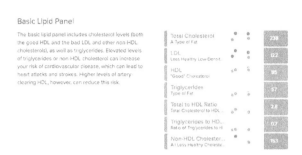

Figure 3. Basic Lipid Panel results from my Advanced Heart Health test through WellnessFX.

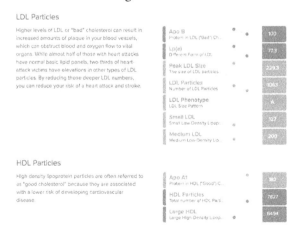

Figure 4. LDL and HDL particle results from my Advanced Heart Health test through WellnessFX.

According to several studies over the past two decades, there is a strong correlation between increased risk of premature heart disease and decreasing size and density of LDL particles. Knowing total LDL only reveals part of the picture. When it comes to cardiovascular risk, higher numbers of smaller, more dense particles indicates an *increased* risk of heart disease compared with lower numbers of these same particles. The overall idea is to have a higher amount of larger, less dense, "fluffy" particles, and to have a lower amount of smaller, more dense particles. The smaller and more dense the particles, the higher the risk of inflammation and blockage in the arteries.

Lipoprotein(a), also known as Lp(a) (pronounced "Lp little a") are specific types of small LDL-like particles that inflame the blood and makes it sticky and prone to clotting, thus increasing your risk of heart attack, stroke, and other cardiovascular problems. Studies show a direct, linear correlation between high Lp(a) in your blood and risk: the higher your Lp(a) cholesterol numbers, the more plaque buildup in your arteries, and the higher your risk of cardiovascular disease.

I'll spare you the exact science of what lipoproteins are made of and how they operate in the bloodstream. But I do encourage you to do more of your own research and, perhaps more importantly, testing to understand what's going on in your heart health picture.

As a reminder, I am not a Medical Doctor. None of this information is intended to be medical advice, but rather to share my personal health journey.

To learn more, I suggest you do your own research: independently online, with your current or new functional medicine physician, or by reading a book about these topics. Both *Cholesterol Clarity* by Jimmy Moore and Dr. Eric Westman and *The Paleo Cardiologist: The Natural Way to Heart Health* by Dr. Jack Wolfson discuss these topics in greater detail.

Not pictured in figure 3 or figure 4, but included in my Advanced Heart Health test, was a measurement of my Omega-3 and Omega-6 levels. I learned my Omega-3 to Omega-6 ratio could be improved, so I've been focusing on eating more Omega-3s from quality sources (like wild salmon and sardines) and avoiding foods higher in Omega-6s (such as grain-fed animal proteins and certain vegetable oils). I've also been supplementing with Omega-3s from Nordic

Naturals, a company who sources very high-quality fish oils, as well as a DHA supplement extracted from algae oil called MitoLife.

The Advanced Heart Health test is just one example of the important tests you can use to learn more about what's going on inside your body. Others to consider include those that help you understand your fatty acid profile, electrolyte levels, vitamin and mineral levels, and vital signs, as well as liver, bone, blood, metabolic, and hormone health.

If you go to https://www.WellnessFX.com you can purchase several different tests, ranging from a $60 Vitamin D test to a $925 Premium test, which will cover nearly all important blood tests.

Do you know your Vitamin D levels?

When I first had my Vitamin D levels tested in April 2015, I had just spent a long, cold winter in Iowa with minimal outdoor exposure to sunlight. As displayed in Figure 5, my Vitamin D levels at that time came in at 50 ng/ml, and the optimal range provided by WellnessFX is 30–100 ng/ml. Though my Vitamin D level was within that optimal range, it was still lower than I wanted it to be.

However, my Vitamin D levels trended upward over the course of a year and a half. I guess that's what moving to California and the occasional proper supplementation can do for you!

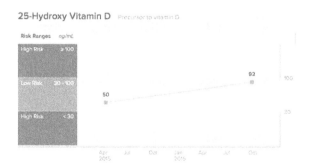

Figure 5. My Vitamin D serum levels from WellnessFX.

As you may notice, Wellness FX's optimal range is 30–100 ng/ml. However, other bodies of research suggest slightly different ranges, such as 35–60 ng/ml. Additionally, research shows having too much Vitamin D in supplement form can do more harm than good. **Make sure you consult a well-qualified health professional and do your own research before choosing what sort of supplementation to do.**

We'll talk more about choosing the right prevention-based holistic health care and wellness teams in the next chapter. Because remember, it's not just important to know your blood work, but to also make sense of it so you can take proper action as needed. In the meantime, here is one quick tip you can act on.

Quick Health Hacker Tip: Organize your blood work.

Do you have any printed copies of past blood work you've received from a doctor? If not, I suggest you could call your doctor or clinic and request this information.

It's not just important to KNOW your blood work, but also to ORGANIZE your information in one place so you can reference it later. That might mean a physical folder with real paper in a cabinet, an electronic file in your Google Drive or Dropbox folder, or it might be stored on another website, like I do through WellnessFX (see Figure 6).

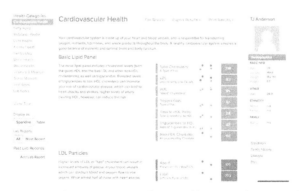

Figure 6. My secure online WellnessFX dashboard.

Starting to organize your blood work in one place, getting regular testing (about once a year), and making a point to research about different, more advanced tests to consider will set you on a path to optimizing your inner, cellular health. And if you already have past blood work on hand, you can create an account with WellnessFX and upload your biomarker results for free.

There are several other advanced lab testing and direct-to-consumer companies you can consider, some of which your doctor may be able to order for you or may be covered by your insurance. Examples include, but are not limited to, SpectraCell, Genova Labs, EveryWell, and InsideTracker.

Now that we have an idea of the importance of advanced blood testing, it's time we transition to the second principle of measuring what matters.

Principle 2: Know Your Genetics

Craig Venter and his team helped sequence the entire human genome in 2001. Genetic testing has grown in popularity ever since, but are we placing too much weight as a country on the importance of testing our genetics? I don't think so.

You see, a lot of people think that genes *control* their destiny. The truth is they don't. They only *influence* our destiny. According to recent research on epigenetics, just because you have a cancer gene doesn't mean it has to be "turned on." As Dr. Andrew Rostenberg, founder of Beyond MTHFR, states on his website: "Not only are our genes powerful, but they are also malleable and programmable—they are never static…you must realize that your genes are not your destiny, but they are your tendency."

Note: In case you're wondering, MTHFR is the acronym given to the enzyme methylenetetrahydrofolate that plays an important role in producing certain amino acids (the building blocks of protein) and is especially vital to converting the amino acid homocysteine into another amino acid, called methionine. It's one of the more important genetic mutations to look for, as it could be responsible for key underlying health issues going on in your life.

Thankfully, with testing available to understand our genetic makeup, we now have the ability to understand potential genetic mutations that may influence our health and make relevant changes to our diet, lifestyle, environment, and supplement regimen to support optimal functioning of our genes.

Involved in this process of hacking our DNA is a key pathway inside of our bodies called the Methylation Cycle. Have you heard of it? I hadn't until I was directed to the work of Dr. Amy Yasko, an expert in biochemistry, molecular biology, and biotechnology. While I haven't met Dr. Yasko, I have started learning from her by reading articles and other content on her website, as well as her book, *Feel Good Nutrigenomics*. This book breaks down the important connection between our nutrition, supplementation strategies, and genetics. It answers the questions: What are the most important parts of genetic data that influence our health? What areas of our health are most impacted by our genetic makeup? The answer? The methylation cycle.

What is the Methylation Cycle and Why is it Important?

According to Dr. Amy Yasko, the **Methylation Cycle** is a biochemical pathway involved in almost every bodily biochemical reaction and occurs billions of times *every second* in our cells. That's why figuring out what's going on in this cycle and, specifically, what genetic mutations one may have that can affect this cycle, can contribute to health optimization and reduced symptoms. According to Dr. Yasko's website, the methylation cycle can affect various bodily functions:

- Detoxification
- Immune function
- Maintaining DNA
- Energy production
- Mood balance
- Controlling inflammation

Each of these processes helps the body respond to environmental stressors, detoxify, adapt, and rebuild. As such, lowered methylation function may contribute to many major chronic conditions:

- Cardiovascular Disease
- Cancer
- Diabetes

- Adult neurological conditions
- Autism and other spectrum disorders
- Chronic Fatigue Syndrome
- Alzheimer's disease
- Miscarriages, fertility, and problems in pregnancy
- Allergies, immune system, and digestive problems
- Mood and psychiatric disorders
- Aging

So what steps do we need to take to fully understand our genetic profile and the potentially important genetic mutations that may be influencing our methylation cycle?

Dr. Yasko offers several different health tests on her website; however, some are quite advanced and are priced accordingly. For example, Dr. Yasko sells her nutrigenomic test for $495 online at http://HolisticHeal.com. This test looks at thirty of the most important single nucleotide polymorphisms (SNPs, pronounced "snips"), how they interact with nutrition and supplements, and how these interactions may assist you in optimizing your genetic functioning. There are three simple, inexpensive steps one can take to get started exploring his or her genetic data.

Step 1: Get Your Raw DNA Sequenced through 23AndMe

With over one million genotyped members worldwide (that is, people who have sequenced their genome), 23andMe is one of the most reputable services for DNA testing on the planet. As some of you may recall, in 2013, 23andMe got into a bit of trouble with the FDA for claiming their tests could be interpreted as medical advice. Well, they no longer provide medical advice; only raw data with a few highlights of important areas to consider.

For example, they provide more than thirty-five Carrier Reports. Being a "carrier" means you carry one genetic variant of a particular condition. According to their website, "Carriers do not typically have the condition, but they can pass a genetic variant down to their children. If both parents are carriers there's a 25 percent chance their child will have the condition."

Now, regardless of whether you're a parent who wants to learn if you have passed or could pass something down to your children or you simply want to understand what's going on with your genes so you can optimize your health and prevent disease, 23andMe is the best place to start.

There are two options on their website for purchase: an Ancestry service, which costs $99, and a Health plus Ancestry service, which costs $199. The Health plus Ancestry service is recommended because it will provide you with a breakdown of raw genetic data and not simply your ancestry information.

It's a pretty simple process. You buy a kit on their website, they ship you the kit, you spit some saliva into a bottle, close it up, and ship it to their lab.

A week or two later, you'll get a notification when they have completed your DNA report and it is ready to download from 23andMe's website.

Step 2: Download Your DNA Report from 23andMe and upload it into a Third-Party Application

Once you have downloaded your DNA report from 23andMe.com, I suggest you wait to review this information. This is your *raw* data, which can be quite confusing to the average person. Based on my research, the standard and recommended practice is to download your DNA Report from 23andMe and upload it into a third-party application to make sense of your DNA information. That's what I did. There are several third-party programs available online:

- **Sterling's App.** A good friend and fellow "hacker" suggested the Sterling's App available online at https://MTHFRsupport.com/sterlings-app/. The app costs $30 and provides a clean way to analyze and understand all of your genetic data. It's pretty simple. You purchase the application, upload raw data from 23andMe, and voilà—your information is uploaded and synthesized into a powerful database with an in-depth analysis of your genetic data.
- **GeneticGenie.org.** I also have personal experience with this service. It's very user-friendly, simply asking for a donation in return for a one page PDF highlighting the most important genes for people to review. Figure 7 displays my Methylation Report from Genetic Genie.

- **LiveWello.com.** I have not tried LiveWello, but they seem to be getting good reviews online. This is another option to consider.

genetic genie

Name: TJ Anderson
Profile: Methylation Profile
Generated: 10/24/2016

Gene & Variation	rsID	Alleles	Result
COMT V158M	rs4680	AG	+/-
COMT H62H	rs4633	CT	+/-
COMT P199P	rs769224	GG	-/-
VDR Bsm	rs1544410	CC	-/-
VDR Taq	rs731236	AA	+/+
MAO A R297R	rs6323	T	+/+
ACAT1-02	rs3741049	GG	-/-
MTHFR C677T	rs1801133	GG	-/-
MTHFR 03 P39P	rs2066470	GG	-/-
MTHFR A1298C	rs1801131	GG	+/+
MTR A2756G	rs1805087	AG	+/-
MTRR A66G	rs1801394	AG	+/-
MTRR H595Y	not found	n/a	not genotyped
MTRR K350A	rs162036	AG	+/-
MTRR R415T	not found	n/a	not genotyped
MTRR A664A	rs1802059	GG	-/-
BHMT-02	rs567754	CC	-/-
BHMT-04	not found	n/a	not genotyped
BHMT-08	rs651852	TT	+/+
AHCY-01	rs819147	TT	-/-

Figure 7. My full Methylation Report, highlighting my genetic mutations.

Of these three options, I personally enjoy my experience with Genetic Genie; however, I suggest you do your own research and consider all three (and potentially others) before making a decision about which program you want to use to analyze your key genetic mutations.

Step 3: Review Your Mutation Analysis, Do Research, and Get Expert Feedback

Information is not necessarily the key—how we artfully make sense of that information so we can take appropriate action is what really matters. After you complete the first two steps, your next step is to understand and make sense of your genetic profile by looking for key genetic mutations. Yes, we're looking for specific SNPs in which a particular gene in your body has gone through some sort of mutation.

Don't worry. It's not as scary as you might think. We all have genetic mutations going on inside our bodies.

Here is the write-up Genetic Genie provided in conjunction with my DNA mutation report to help me understand the basics prior to learning what my particular mutations meant:

Genetic Genie Methylation Profile Analysis

Although mutations can occur at any time during our lifetime, it is most likely we are born with these mutations and will have them throughout our life. These inherited mutations have been passed down to us from previous generations (our parents and grandparents) and may be passed to future generations (our children). This may be an explanation as to why certain traits or diseases "run in the family."

Although we cannot change our genetic code, we can change how our genes are expressed. Research has revealed that our gene expression is not determined solely by hereditary factors, but it is also influenced by our diet, nutritional status, toxic load and environmental influences or stressors. This phenomenon has been termed "epigenetics." Researchers in the growing field of epigenetics have demonstrated that certain genes can be over—or under-expressed with certain disease processes. Researchers in this field hope that by understanding of how these genes are regulated and what is influencing them, we may be able to change their expression. Using epigenetic concepts along with a good understanding of the methylation cycle, researchers have begun to make recommendations to optimize genetic expression and help to restore health.

Disclaimer: The information on this website is for entertainment and informational purposes only and should not be used a substitute for a consultation with a health care provider. You, the reader, are instructed to consult with a qualified health care provider prior to acting on any suggestions presented on this website. This information is not intended for the diagnosis, treatment or cure of disease.

Genetic Genie went on to provide a complete six-page analysis of my key genetic mutations and what that means to me, which was very helpful. But per their advice, I also consulted with my naturopath who helped guide me in optimizing my genetics.

Now you might be wondering, what exactly did I learn? And, perhaps more importantly, what changes did I make in my lifestyle based on this information?

The truth is, I'm still in the process of hacking—that is, making applicable changes in my lifestyle based on my genetic information. I'll spare you all of the details, but for now, here are highlights of my key mutations and how I am addressing them:

- **I have one MTHFR homozygous mutation, MTHFR A1298C.**
  - o In consulting with my naturopath, she suggested I include a methylfolate supplement to support this mutation as well as methyl B12.
  - o I had already started taking a supplement called Qualia from Neurohacker Collective, which included the methyl B12 my body required. So I stuck with this supplement, added methylfolate, and started cycling on and off of both.

    Note: I'll share more about Qualia in Act 5. It's one of my favorite supplements, acting as a multi-vitamin for my brain that delivers a nice boost in focus, mental clarity, and overall energy.

- **I also have another important gene mutation, COMT.**
  - o Due to my COMT mutation, my naturopath suggested that I try consuming both niacin and magnesium, two crucial nutrients that can help the body adapt to and better use the methylfolate and methyl B12 in the overall methylation cycle.

After I received this report, I did a bit more research to understand what to do moving forward. I also found specialized health professionals who are trained and well-versed in supporting patients with this type of information. (We'll talk more about designing your own health care and wellness team in chapter 12.) Perhaps most importantly, I took my complete health picture into consideration and kept testing and tracking other important information to understand what could be going on in my health.

For example, I learned that I had a VDR-Taq homozygous mutation. This particular mutation may impact my ability to properly process Vitamin D. And we all know how important Vitamin D is to our health and energy, as well as our ability to prevent disease and live a high quality of life on this planet. In fact, optimal Vitamin D levels can slash your risk of cancer by as much as 60 percent, according to some studies.

One well-respected integrative physician, Dr. Joseph Mercola of www. Mercola.com, talks a lot about the role of Vitamin D and how it's actually much more than a vitamin:

> While scientists refer to Vitamin D as a vitamin, it is actually a steroid hormone obtained from sun exposure, food sources, and supplementation. Common types of Vitamin D are Vitamin D2 and D3. Compared with D2, Vitamin D3 is 87 percent more effective, and is the preferred form for addressing insufficient levels of Vitamin D.

Understanding the role Vitamin D plays in our overall health picture is vitally important. It's much more than just another vitamin. But we also need to take an individualized approach to understanding current serum blood levels of Vitamin D in our bodies and whether we may have a genetic mutation that impacts our metabolism of Vitamin D.

Have you ever received a blood test and questioned the results? When I first got my Vitamin D blood levels back and learned they were borderline low I wondered why.

Was it the winter weather causing this? Could there be other factors? Were the results even correct? Thankfully I stumbled upon my Vitamin D receptor mutation in my Genetic Genie analysis to help put the pieces together. The relationship between these two factors suggested the results may be correct, but I wanted to dig a bit deeper to confirm my hypothesis. That's what led me to the third principle of measuring what matters—knowing your micronutrients.

Principle 3: Know Your Micronutrients

When it comes to measuring what matters, I would be remiss if I didn't mention nutrition. There are a few key tests I recommend that can result in a significant upgrade in our health, such as a food sensitivity test or microbiome (gut health) test, but for the purposes of this section we will focus on the Micronutrient Deficiency test.

When I was living in San Diego in 2016, I had the opportunity to spend a lot of time around some naturopathic doctors in advanced preventative health clinics. I had just visited the ER back in Iowa, and didn't really have a great sense that my health care team was providing me with all the best testing and resources to help me optimize my health. Simply put, I was hungry to learn more about what was going on in my health. That led me to consider seeing new doctors who didn't just tell me general health information or how to manage a certain symptom. I wanted and needed to find doctors who understood how to approach lifestyle change in concert with lab work. I also wanted to learn about new advanced blood tests that were available—blood tests that didn't just say whether or not I was healthy, but that allowed me to build a precise plan to tweak my nutrition and supplementation in a way that was specific to what was going on inside my body.

Micronutrient Test by SpectraCell

I learned about one specific test that could help support me in this area—the Micronutrient Test (MNT). When it comes to micronutrient optimization, knowing what to eat without proper testing is very difficult. This test, which has been proven to provide the most accurate analysis of micronutrient deficiencies, measures the function of thirty-five nutritional components, including vitamins, antioxidants, minerals, and amino acids.

Most diagnostic and risk assessment tests are based on measurements of static levels of certain nutrients in serum, which are not always the best indicators for assessing cell metabolism and utilization. For example, you can get a serum Vitamin D 25 hydroxy test, which provides a snapshot of the current level of Vitamin D in your body. But this test doesn't look at your body's reserve level of this important vitamin or your body's ability to use it. SpectraCell's MNT does. The MNT is a functional test measuring thirty-five components on an *intracellular level.*

What specifically does the test measure?

- Vitamins (A, B1, B2, B3, B6, B12, Biotin, Folate, Pantothenate, C, D, and K)
- Minerals (Calcium, Magnesium, Manganese, Zinc, and Copper)
- Amino Acids (Asparagine, Glutamine, and Serine)
- Fatty Acids (Oleic Acid)
- Antioxidants (Alpha Lipoic Acid, Coenzyme Q10, Cysteine, Glutathione, Selenium, and Vitamin E)
- Carbohydrate Metabolism (Chromium, Fructose Sensitivity, and Glucose-Insulin Metabolism)
- Metabolites (Choline, Inositol, and Carnitine)
- SPECTROX for total antioxidant function
- IMMUNIDEX Immune Response Score

What will you see and learn?

When I got my SpectraCell MNT report back, it was pretty user-friendly. The lab results included an overview page with all deficiencies listed, including numerical data and clean graphic reports easily showing areas of deficiency as well as repletion and supplementation recommendations.

I was able to review my results with a good friend, Kirstin Keilty, who has her master of science degree in human nutrition and is a Certified Nutrition Specialist. Kirstin, who works for SpectraCell as a clinical nutrition consultant, helps doctors and patients across the country understand how to read tests like the MNT. And she definitely helped me change how I look at nutrition with one simple statement: **"Nutrition is a concert—not a solo."**

In other words, if one micronutrient, such as glutathione, is low, we don't need to simply supplement with glutathione. There are several other micronutrients and lab markers that contribute to levels being low. We need to look at our nutrition and micronutrients as a concert, with multiple singers individually singing different notes. Each voice (and each nutrient) can affect the others indirectly.

All things considered, I learned I was doing pretty well, but I did have a few key deficiencies to consider improving through targeted nutrition, supplementation, and lifestyle habits. Figure 8 includes a snapshot of my results.

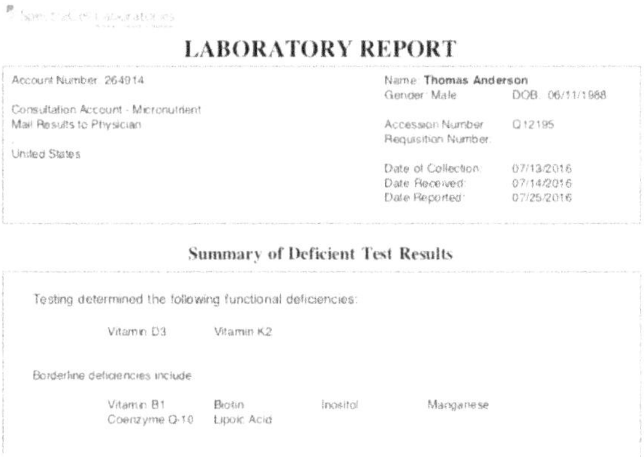

LABORATORY REPORT

Account Number: 264914

Consultation Account - Micronutrient
Mail Results to Physician

United States

Name: Thomas Anderson
Gender: Male   DOB: 06/11/1988

Accession Number   Q12195
Requisition Number

Date of Collection: 07/13/2016
Date Received: 07/14/2016
Date Reported: 07/25/2016

Summary of Deficient Test Results

Testing determined the following functional deficiencies:

    Vitamin D3   Vitamin K2

Borderline deficiencies include:

    Vitamin B1   Biotin   Inositol   Manganese
    Coenzyme Q-10 Lipoic Acid

Figure 8. My lab results highlighting my primary and borderline deficiencies.

As you can see, I was deficient in Vitamin D3 and Vitamin K2, two fat-soluble vitamins crucial for optimal health and proper cellular function. And I was borderline in a few other areas.

If you recall, I have a homozygous Vitamin D receptor mutation, which, after analyzing my results with SpectraCell, could be playing a role in my Vitamin D levels. Additionally, after reviewing my lifestyle changes over the past two years (including my large increase in the macronutrient fat) with my naturopathic doctor, we determined that my body (and specifically my liver) might still be getting used to processing higher fat levels and fat-soluble vitamins.

This has led me to supplement with Vitamin D (up to 5,000–10,000 IU's daily), supplement with K2, and increase certain foods to help assist my body in producing and creating a nice flow of bile through my liver, which plays a direct role in my ability to process fat-soluble vitamins.

When I first did this, I was a bit overwhelmed. I had no idea what I was doing and relied on conversations with people who were smarter than me on this topic as well as my own research to understand how to best move forward. That's important—surround yourself with the right people, technology, and resources to make sense of your health information. Remember to view your nutrition as a concert and not a solo. And develop the hunger, as a health-conscious consumer, to want to measure and learn about what's going on in your health.

While genetic information is something we may only check once (it won't necessarily change throughout our life), measuring blood work and micronutrient levels can be measured on a regular basis, perhaps once a year, depending on how closely you want to monitor any lifestyle changes you are making.

Principle 4: Know Your Heart Rate Variability

There is one more principle I want to touch on that you can measure on a daily basis. It's non-invasive and may be more important than anything else you're measuring right now.

As we discussed earlier, expanding our awareness and action in our breathing is integral to managing our stress. But is there a way to actually measure the quality of our breathing so we can quantifiably take our health to the next level?

For the past few years, I've been using a Heart Rate Variability (HRV) device and application on my phone called The Inner Balance. Developed by an organization called HeartMath Inc., the Inner Balance analyzes and displays the rhythm of our heart, measured by HRV. HeartMath has over 25 years of experience in understanding HRV, which has been the subject of more than 250 independent, peer-reviewed studies.

What exactly is HRV? HRV is a way of assessing variation in the time interval between heartbeats, or the beat-to-beat interval. Decreased variability has been identified as a marker of increased pathology and as a predictor of morbidity and mortality in multiple medical disciplines. Meaning if you have low HRV, it could put you at slightly higher risk for a heart attack, stroke, or other physiological phenomenon that may lead to an early death.

So, how can you start measuring your HRV? Download HeartMath's Inner Balance app and purchase their Inner Balance device.

The Inner Balance by HeartMath

How exactly does this Inner Balance device work? One end of the device plugs into your phone and the other end has a sensor that attaches to your ear to measure your HRV. HRV levels show how emotional states are affecting our nervous system moment to moment, which allows us to improve the quality of communication between our heart and brain through relaxed, intentional, heart-centered breathing. With this sort of self-generated, real-time feedback loop, we can use our breath and thoughts to help manage our stress and build more resilience in our lives.

Figure 9 provides a glimpse at what an actual Inner Balance session looks like. At the top of the far left panel, you'll notice the HRV line changing over time. In the lower part of the far left panel, you'll see a real-time feedback loop that allows you to track how well you're doing within a particular session. Just as a personal trainer or fitness instructor can provide real-time feedback on your form during workouts, so can this innovative device and app. The Inner Balance technology trains us to create a healthy and efficient physiological state called HRV coherence, when HRV and breathing rhythms are in sync.

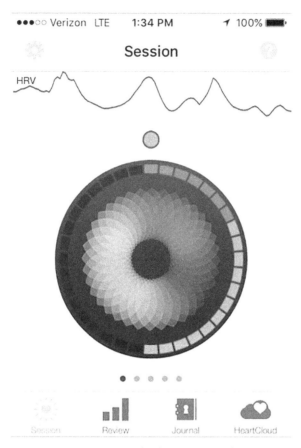

Figure 9. Inside the HeartMath app.

As displayed in figure 9, green represents high HRV coherence, blue represents medium HRV coherence, and red represents low HRV coherence. So if you think about something that conjures a positive emotion, your breathing rhythms will have high coherence with your HRV. And if you think about something that is more stressful, your breathing rhythms will have low coherence with your HRV. Thanks to this technology, I've noticed just taking a break in my day to settle down and get feedback on my breath and how my thoughts impact my emotions and body can be very powerful. It's a reminder not just to breathe, but to focus on *how* we breathe—through our hearts in a mindful and loving way.

But don't just take my word for it. Even biohacking leaders are using this technology to assess their stress. As Dave Asprey shares,

When you use this little game and you breathe in and you breathe out, you realize to make it turn green you have to also think about something positive like puppies to conjure an emotion like happiness, peace, or gratitude. And if you do you'll notice, oh, my emotions change the way my heart beats. Not by changing the number of beats per minute, but by changing the spacing between the heart beats.

The middle panel of figure 9 provides data from past sessions. You'll see a percentage breakdown for each of my levels of coherence. Within the app, you're also able to adjust the difficulty level and receive points for your progress. (Who doesn't like a little gamification of our health?!)

The far right panel of figure 9 shows a real-time analysis of a session, showing a graphical view of my HRV over the course of the session.

Isn't it interesting how technology can both contribute to increasing our stress and also support us as we attempt to reduce our stress? While the Inner Balance may not be essential to life, it is a very powerful tool that can assist you in assessing your stress and training your brain and heart how to interact with each other—a powerful area of potential for the human species to address.

If there's one health app I recommend, it's the Inner Balance by HeartMath.

In Review

We just covered four key principles to follow when looking to measure success in our health. And you might be wondering, "Aren't there a lot of other important things to measure (e.g., your overall amount and type of body fat, sleep data, or blood pressure)?"

Well, yes, there is value in knowing these types of markers as well. But my intention is to highlight some of the recent information and approaches I've focused on to optimize my health for the long term—strategies and technology that you may not have seen or heard of yet.

I hope this section was helpful for you to understand what else might be possible to learn and measure about your health. The next step is making sense of this information with the help of your personal health care team, which we'll discuss in the next chapter.

Summary:

- Consider tracking and organizing your blood work and key medical and health history information to know more about what's going on inside your body.
- Seek to understand your blood work and don't just rely on what your doctor says.
- Consider getting advanced lab testing from a company like WellnessFX or SpectraCell.
- Genetics play a big role in your health, but you still have an opportunity to influence them.
- There are new biomarkers, like Heart Rate Variability (HRV), that are thought to affect overall mortality that you may want to begin measuring in your day-to-day life.

Action Items:

1. How did this chapter resonate with you? Did it get you thinking about some important areas of your health to measure?
2. Put your blood work data online—either a simple spreadsheet or a website like https://www.WellnessFX.com (a great free resource for you to upload your lab results online).
3. Consider reading *Cholesterol Clarity* by Jimmy Moore and Dr. Eric Westman or *The Paleo Cardiologist* by Dr. Jack Wolfson. These are great books to read if you'd like to dive a bit deeper into understanding research about what real heart health looks like.
4. Purchase Inner Balance from HeartMath and start experimenting with intentional, HRV breathwork to increase your resilience and manage your stress more effectively.

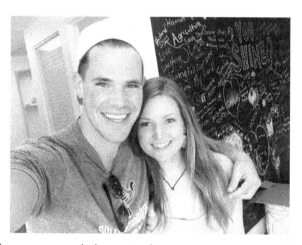

With my naturopath doctor, Katherine, in San Diego, California.

CHAPTER 12

How to Build Your Health Care Team:

The Power of Clear Direction and Accountability

Functional medicine is about causes, not symptoms. It is getting to the root of the problem.
– Mark Hyman, MD

When I left the ER in February 2016, I had no answers. I never saw a doctor while I was in the ER and never heard any details about what was going on in my health.

All I was told was, "You're stable."

Thankfully I took an active role in my health at this time and tried to schedule a visit with my doctor the next day. Not surprisingly, my doctor had no time, but I was able to see an Advanced Registered Nurse Practitioner (ARNP). During this visit, we went over my "episode," as I was calling it, as well as my lab work from the ER, which showed a clearer picture of what was going on inside my body.

We analyzed all of the key lab numbers to see what was going on, only to find out I had an electrolyte issue.

At 129 mmol/L, my sodium levels were dangerously low. The optimal range is supposed to be 135–145 mmol/L. My potassium and chloride were both a bit low as well, but the most concerning level was sodium.

"Just drink Gatorade and eat some salty foods," she said.

You bet. Thanks for the smart, healthy tip (sigh).

After two weeks of eating more hydrating foods and consuming more high-quality sea salt and quality spring water (filled with essential minerals), my sodium levels went back up and everything had normalized.

But I never would have known that if I hadn't followed up with my health care team for help and guidance in comparing my before and after blood work.

The future of health care is a proactive, predictive, and personalized practice of medicine that empowers people to take an active role in their health. And if you want the best outcomes, you need to ask for help and choose the best doctor and health care team that work for you and your goals.

Ask For Help

When I started my intentional health hacker journey in 2013, I had no roadmap or blueprint, but still thought I knew what I was doing. More specifically, I didn't know how to best access the health care system. And if I am being honest, I was scared. I didn't want to ask for help. I thought I knew enough about myself and my health to manage it myself. Or at least I thought I could find the information I needed online. Boy, was I wrong. I was overwhelmed and didn't want to admit I didn't know something about my health. I didn't want to ask for help. Fast-forward to today, and that's all changed—dramatically.

Asking for help takes courage, but it also takes the intention to ask for help from the right people.

Building our own health care team is not something we often consider as consumers. We don't always realize what's possible and how much power and choice we really have. On one hand, having an overwhelming number of choices can be just that—overwhelming. On the other hand, having the ability to choose your own doctor and entire health care team can be quite freeing. Especially

when you're confident you have highly competent professionals who know a lot about the human body and the power it has to heal naturally.

In this chapter, we will explore the different types of doctors and health care practitioners you can consider when building your health care team. We'll discuss the differences between functional, allopathic, and naturopathic medicine. And we'll begin to understand how to build a health care team trained in partnering with you in your care—addressing your whole body and lifestyle goals, not simply a set of symptoms.

The goal is to build a team and an approach that is cost-effective, time-sensitive, and focused on powerful, quality outcomes. So let's get started.

How do we build our own health care team?

As discussed in chapter 1, our traditional health care system in the US is mostly a sick-care system. It's largely driven by the pathogenic model, where professionals are trained to understand and focus on the origin and treatment of disease, not necessarily to support health optimization, well-being, and the creation of health-ease.

Lucky for us, there are several growing movements in alternative, holistic care that actually address causes and not just symptoms. With a balance between salutogenesis and pathogenesis, integrative and functional medicine are leading the way, providing an opportunity to understand what this means for us as health care consumers.

Functional Medicine—The Future of Health Care

In spring 2016, I attended the Institute for Functional Medicine's (IFM) Annual International Conference in San Diego. Surrounded by hundreds of holistic-minded and functionally trained health professionals, I was in heaven. You see, I had just spent the past year designing health coach trainings for large health care systems across the country, many of which were behind the eight ball in their approach to supporting patients with lifestyle change. I knew there was a growing movement of alternative, functional, and integrative medicine spreading like wildfire, and I was smack dab in the middle of it. The IFM conference represents functional medicine at its best—hyperbaric chamber here, heart rate variability measurements there, nutrigenomics testing, micronutrient testing, heavy metal detox companies, light therapy companies, professional-grade supplement companies—you name it, it was there.

I was at this event on behalf of The Rejuvenation Station, providing on-site nutrient IV therapy for attendees of major conferences and events. I had just started consulting for the two naturopathic doctors who co-own this business and I was excited to get a taste of this industry. During this event, something clicked for me. The conversations I had, the speakers I listened to, and the energy at the event resulted in an overall experience that was quite profound.

As I spoke with different vendor organizations and health professionals, my perspective of our health care system started to shift. Here were all of these companies and health professionals advancing their knowledge, connections, and experience for one sole purpose—to advance the health outcomes of patients (what some health professionals now refer to as clients, customers, or even health participants). This was the future of health care.

What Exactly is Functional Medicine?

According to the IFM, the Functional Medicine model is defined as "an individualized, patient-centered, science-based approach that empowers patients and practitioners to work together to address the underlying causes of disease and promote optimal wellness."

The goal of functional medicine trained practitioners is clear—to understand the root cause or causes of a person's disease and symptoms and take the time necessary to approach the patient as a whole, not to simply try to fix the hole (the symptoms).

Put simply, functional medicine is about taking our health to the next level. And realizing we're not alone. We can work in collaboration with a team to support us in our journey.

The tree and soil graphic from chapter 2 is a great reminder of all the factors that play a role in one's symptoms or current state of health.

Now that we have a deeper understanding of what a true pathogenic model (focused on treating the cause or causes and not just the symptoms) looks like, it's time to dive into a philosophical approach that pervades western medicine and plays a role in how physicians approach the disease process.

The Role of Reductionism—Focusing on a Single Factor

Most conventional medicine today is based on a **reductionist approach**, characterized by reducing complex interactions and entities to the sum of their parts in order to make them easier to study. While a reductionist or allopathic approach has a place in medicine (and might make sense to you right now), it's a strategy that doesn't always work out.

To understand more about the role of reductionism in medicine, let's explore some research presented by authors Ahn, Tewari, Poon, and Phillips in two *Public Library of Science (PLOS) Medicine* journal articles. In the first article, "The Limits of Reductionism in Medicine: Could Systems Biology Offer an Alternative?" the authors review the history of reductionism in medicine and the role it plays today, as well as provide an overview of the value of taking a systems-biology approach in clinical medicine.

There is a deeply held belief inside the practice of reductionism that each disease has one single target for medical treatment. For example, for an infection, the target is the pathogen, and for cancer, the tumor, so on and so forth. You get the point. While this approach has resulted in some success, it leaves little room for contextual information. As explained by Ahn et al.,

> A young immunocompromised man with pneumococcal pneumonia usually gets the same antibiotic treatment as an elderly woman with the same infection. The disease, and not the person affected by it, becomes the central focus. Our contemporary analytical tools are simply not designed to address more complex questions, and, thus, questions such as "how do a person's sleeping habits, diet, living condition, comorbidities, and stress collectively contribute to his/her heart disease?" remain largely unanswered.

An alternative approach to addressing these complex questions has been receiving recent attention—the systems perspective. In the same article, Ahn et al. go on to say,

> Rather than dividing a complex problem into its component parts, the systems perspective appreciates the holistic and composite characteristics of a problem and evaluates the problem with the use of computational and mathematical tools. The systems perspective is rooted in the assumption that the forest cannot be explained by studying the trees individually.

The Need for an Integrative Approach

While reading through these thought-provoking articles, I realized that reductionism need not be tossed out entirely. In fact, it has a place in approaching certain types of disease. However, we, as a society, need to understand which diseases are best approached from a reductionist perspective versus a systems-oriented perspective. In the second article of the series, Ahn et al. discuss how complex chronic diseases are better addressed by an integrative approach:

> In clinical medicine, complex, chronic diseases such as diabetes, coronary artery disease, or asthma are examples where this rule may apply. In these examples, a single factor is rarely implicated as solely responsible for disease development or presentation. Rather, multiple factors are often identified, and the disease evolves through complex interactions between them. Consequently, a perspective in which the interactions and dynamics are centrally integrated into the analytical methods may be better suited. Systems perspectives, unlike reductionists, focus on these interrelationships and, therefore, may be the optimal method for complex chronic diseases.

In short, reductionism often fails us by leading us to believe there is only one solution to a problem. Reductionism seems to become less effective when it fails to take into account important information, such as lifestyle habits or environmental toxicities, which could play a role in a patient's health or disease.

Judging by the information in this field of research, some of our most important issues are more appropriately addressed using a systems-oriented approach.

Understanding the fundamental differences between these two approaches to health care and medicine is important, but not always easy, for us as health hacking consumers. If we believe in the value of taking an integrative, whole-person, systems-oriented approach, we need to consider which doctors to include on our team and for what purpose.

The first step to building your health care team is finding the right doctor or doctors, preferably who value the philosophy of functional medicine—treating the cause and not just the symptoms—to support us in our salutogenic, self-care model of health.

What follows is a list of some of the most common types of doctors in the US today and why you might consider working with each.

Medical Doctors (MDs)

Traditionally, Medical Doctors (MDs) are trained in an allopathic approach to health care, focused on combating disease with interventions like pharmaceuticals and surgery, rather than lifestyle. MDs are incredibly smart human beings and very important to our health care system; however, most MDs' expertise is not in prevention or using lifestyle measures to reverse or prevent disease. While some MDs might be trained in functional or integrative medicine, most are trained to treat symptoms and not address the root causes.

Why would I consider working with a MD?

I would want an MD to be on my team if I was in need of surgery or had a major illness or sickness (e.g., cancer) and wanted a second opinion. If an MD seemed to understand and have training in nutrition and disease prevention (i.e., studied or trained in functional or integrative medicine) I would consider working with them as my general practitioner as well.

Doctors of Osteopathic Medicine (DOs)

DOs are growing in popularity in our country, and for a good reason. According to the American Association of Osteopathy (AOA), DOs are trained in a whole-person approach. They receive special training in the musculoskeletal system—your body's interconnected system of nerves, muscles, and bones. My sister is a DO and I'm a big fan of this profession—especially DOs who receive extra training in nutrition or functional medicine, and who use a holistic approach with their patients.

Why would I consider working with a DO?

I would work with a DO as my general practitioner if they have advanced training in nutrition or functional medicine and could help me optimize my lab work and genetic information.

Naturopathic Doctors (NDs or NMDs)

NDs (or NMDs) are also growing in popularity due to their training in nutrition, homeopathy, and other lifestyle-based areas to support a patient in healing naturally. According to the American Association of Naturopathic Physicians (AANP), NDs combine the wisdom of nature with the rigors of modern-day science. I personally have several good ND friends, one of which has become my personal doctor. Unfortunately, Naturopathic Doctors are not able to legally practice in every state. At the time of this writing, there are sixteen states (and four provinces in Canada) that allow the practice of naturopathic medicine: Alaska, Arizona, British Columbia, California, Connecticut, Hawaii, Idaho, Kansas, Maine, Manitoba, Minnesota, Montana, New Hampshire, North Dakota, Ontario, Oregon, Saskatchewan, Utah, Vermont, and Washington.

For example, in my home state of Iowa, it is illegal for an ND to practice solely as an ND as well. Crazy, right? Why? Politics and money, my friends. Other professional organizations lobby against naturopathic care becoming legal in their state for several reasons, not the least of which are perceived competition and stigma surrounding the philosophy of this approach.

Why would I consider working with a ND?

I currently work with a ND to help support me with the advanced lab testing services highlighted in chapter 11. For lifestyle management, disease prevention, and health optimization, NDs are one of my top choices.

I personally like working with naturopaths or functional and integrative medicine-trained practitioners. Not just because they are trained in the aforementioned systems approach, but also because they seem to know more and care more about science-based lifestyle behaviors like nutrition and supplementation and how those topics relate to the biochemistry of advanced diagnostic lab testing.

Doctors of Chiropractic Medicine (DCs)

DCs are another option to consider as your general practitioner. I have a lot of friends whose go-to practitioner is a chiropractor, especially if that chiropractor is trained in functional medicine and nutrition. A lot of DCs use diagnostic imaging tools like x-ray to see what's going on with a person while also striving to be holistic-minded. But not all DCs have the capacity to support patients with optimizing their lab work and addressing genetic factors.

Why would I consider working with a DC?

I see a chiropractor on occasion if I feel like my spine is out of alignment or if I have some sort of nerve pain in my neck. (I had an accident in college as a mascot that has resulted in recurrent nerve pain down my arm from a C6-C7 bulged disk.) I view quality DCs (those who treat to solve issues, not to sell you packages that you don't necessarily need) as great members of a health care team to utilize from time to time. Especially the ones who are holistic-minded.

Doctors of Physical Therapy (PTs)

PTs are another great option to consider as a member of your care team. I've worked for Breakthrough Physical Therapy Marketing, an organization supporting the evolution of the private practice physical therapy industry, for the past 12 months, while writing this book. Plus, my brother-in-law is a physical therapist and has treated me successfully a few times. I've seen the power that a PT can have to help someone rehab an injury and get back on their feet.

With millions of Americans experiencing back pain at any given time, physical therapists provide a much alternative to surgery or pain medication.

Why would I consider working with a PT?

I would see (and have seen) a physical therapist if I am experiencing pain, injury, or my body was out of alignment. Physical therapy could be an alternative or compliment to chiropractic care as well. I will see a PT on occasion if I'm experiencing tendonitis or other pain in forearm, elbow, or hand. My body usually responds very well to soft-tissue immobilization for tendonitis in my hands, wrist, neck and other areas, which physical therapists are well equipped to provide. For example, both my local PT in Boulder, Colorado, and my brother-in-law back home in Iowa have helped ease a lot of the pain in my wrist and arm and break up scar tissue with soft-tissue immobilization tools, such as Astym therapy or the previously mentioned Wave Tool.

My Ideal Health and Fitness Team

So what does the ideal health and fitness team look like? I had a chance to sit down with Ben Greenfield, top health and fitness influencer, to discuss this very question. In addition to his wildly informative and at times humorous podcast, Greenfield is also the author of the book *Beyond Training* and has a lot of experience in the health, fitness, and medical communities. According to Greenfield,

> There are three things to look at. First, you want someone who is well-versed in biochemistry, specifically when it comes to optimizing health. Second, you want someone who can think naturally, but also accepts some form of modern medicine who you're able to turn to when you do get sick and need that acute care. And finally, third, you want that person who can take care of you biomechanically. In my opinion, those are the main people you'd want as part of your team. And of course the fourth person is just YOU—there is so much you can manage yourself.

So it turns out we don't just need a doctor to provide acute care as our primary care physician. If we want to build the ideal health and fitness team, we might want to identify team members who specialize specifically in biochemistry and biomechanics.

Here are the main members of my health and fitness team on a monthly or yearly basis:

- **Naturopath/Functional Medicine-Trained Physician** (i.e., my biochemistry doctor with extensive training in nutrition who helps to review my blood, stool, and genetic tests)
- **Movement Specialist** (i.e., my biomechanical trainer, such a functional movement coach or Pilates instructor, who helps focus my physical training efforts toward areas of my body that are weak or impaired)
- **Chiropractor/Physical Therapist** (i.e., my biomechanical doctors who help adjust my physical body when it gets out of alignment or I am experiencing pain)
- **Myself** (Health Hacker/Self Coach)

In the end, it's about rounding out your own customized health care team based on your health and the skill sets and therapies you need to support your path to health optimization.

Three Steps to Choosing Your Health Care Team

1. Do your Research.

Find a primary care doctor or multiple doctors who treat you and your body as a WHOLE, and not just your symptoms. Find someone who is trained in functional medicine, has a background in nutrition, and understands the value and application of alternative, holistic medicine.

You can research doctors in your area, or you can even work with doctors outside of your hometown. One of my friends and naturopathic doctors, Dr. Katherine Zagone, is based out of San Diego, and we often have virtual conversations via email, phone, or video conference call to go over my blood work and talk about my nutrition and supplement game plan. I've connected her with several of my clients, friends, and family members over the last few years, and she remains an option if you are interested.

Another great online resource for finding a functional medicine practitioner is https://www.ifm.org/.

Note: If you are constrained by your insurance and the requirement to stay "in-network," start by looking at your insurance company's website. It's at least worth looking into.

2. Ask Questions.

Have an initial visit with a prospective doctor or a staff member over the phone or via email. It's important to gather key information by asking good questions before selecting your doctor of choice. Here are some questions you could ask:

- How would you describe your practice?
- What therapies do you use? For example, what sort of first-line treatment options do you offer, including diet, herbs, nutritional supplementation, or other lifestyle strategies?
- What kind of lab work do you use (e.g., urine, stool, saliva, or blood tests) to support your understanding of what's going on in my health?
- How do you think you could help me with this particular medical issue that I am experiencing?

For more examples of questions you can ask and what to expect when working with a Functional Medicine practitioner, visit https://www.ifm.org/functional-medicine/patient-resource-center/.

3. Make a Decision.

At the end of the day, regardless of where you're at now in your health, you have an opportunity to make a decision about how you access the health care system and build the holistic health care team you want to build. The freedom to choose your doctor may not be a freedom you were always aware of, but hopefully now you are. Ideally, we would make decisions about our health based on the type of doctor we want to help build our health care strategy, not on our current type of health insurance coverage. As you build your health care team in the next few months or years, continue to ask for help, feedback, and second opinions. This can help you make the most informed and intentional decisions possible in your quest for optimal health and disease prevention.

Health Insurance Alternative—Medical Bill Sharing

In December 2016, when everyone was frantically talking about how to move forward with the health insurance open enrollment period under the Affordable Care Act, I received a notice in the mail about my health insurance policy automatically renewing with a large health insurance company in Iowa.

My premium was going to go from $209 per month to $317 per month—a more than $100 increase for something I hardly use and doesn't keep me healthy in the first place. Not so fast. Instead of renewing my policy, I made the decision to ditch traditional health insurance and try out an alternative—medical bill sharing with an organization called Medi-Share.

What is Medi-Share and how does it work?

Medi-Share is a Health Care Sharing Ministry program that operates similar to health insurance, but often at a lower cost. Each month, your monthly share (or premium) is matched with other members' eligible medical bills. Medi-Share publishes the bills eligible for sharing and coordinates the medical cost sharing between members. In my experience, Medi-Share will email you letting you know the bills to which your monthly share was applied. It's important to note Medi-Share does not promise to pay all medical bills. For example, God forbid you have a life-threatening disease such as cancer and you meet your deductible (known as the Annual Household Portion), your excess medical bills are not guaranteed to be covered; however, according to the Medi-Share website and multiple Medi-Share representatives, members have shared in *every* eligible medical bill published for sharing since 1993 when Medi-Share was created.

Does it meet the requirements of the Affordable Care Act?

Yes, it does. According to the Medi-Share website, members of Health Care Sharing Ministries, like Medi-Share, are exempt from the law and do not face penalties for not purchasing traditional insurance.

Medi-Share Cost and Savings

I previously had a high-deductible traditional health insurance plan, paying a little more than $200 per month with a $5,000 deductible. When I joined Medi-Share (with a high-deductible plan), my premium was $74 per month ($69 plus a $5 service charge).

Instead of paying an extra $108 per month, I *saved* an extra $243 per month. **That's a total of $2,916 in savings per year.** I use that few thousand dollars in annual savings on more prevention-based services, like eating healthy food, exploring different parts of the earth, as well as paying for self-care services like massage, float tanks, and more blood work.

Medi-Share prices are based on how many family members are applying for membership and the date of birth of the oldest applicant. You can choose from various levels of coverage depending on your budget, level of risk, and how you approach your health. If you believe in your ability to avoid major medical needs by focusing on living a healthy lifestyle with less stress and more prevention, you can elect a higher annual household portion or deductible. That's what I did.

Medi-Share also provides a very safe and loving community for fellow Medi-Share members to pray for you in times of poor health. Every month, I get an email letting me know how my monthly share went to support fellow members and their medical bills.

Medi-Share is not for everyone. There are some restrictions; for example, you must identify with being a Christian. Additionally, to receive the most coverage and savings possible, you must use their approved list of PPO providers, which may or may not be trained in functional medicine.

Do I know everything will work out perfectly with Medi-Share? Nope. I'm taking a calculated risk. And I'm going to use this as an experiment to see how I can strategically invest part of my health insurance savings to both improve my health and prevent poor health outcomes from happening in the first place. The bottom line is that alternatives to traditional insurance exist and provide more and more options to consumers.

We all have the power to choose our health future today by building a team and plan rooted in prevention and intention.

Summary:

- There is a difference between allopathic, functional, and naturopathic medicine, and a place for each in health care.
- Most health conditions are more complex than the symptoms we experience.
- A rise in functional, integrative, and naturopathic medicine practitioners is paving the way for vibrant, optimal health for their patients.
- We have the power to interview and choose our own doctor and our entire health care team. It just takes a little bit of research and the courage to ask questions.
- Traditional health insurance is not our only option. There are alternative programs, such as medical bill sharing programs (like Medi-Share), which can help you save money and be part of a supportive, prayer-filled community.

Action Items:

1. What have you learned about how doctors and health professionals are trained differently and how that training may influence their ability to support your health?
2. How do you pay for health insurance? If you're concerned about the cost versus coverage, do some research on alternative options, such as medical bill sharing from organizations like Medi-Share.
3. Build your health care team. Start a list of the health and wellness professionals or therapies you currently utilize or would be interested in utilizing in the future.
4. Follow three steps to choosing your own functional-medicine-minded, primary care doctor:
   - Do Your Research

- Ask Questions
- Make a Decision

Note: If you currently have a doctor and are questioning their level of support and guidance, follow these same three steps to ensure you have the right physician in your corner.

The Health Hacker Process and Game Plan

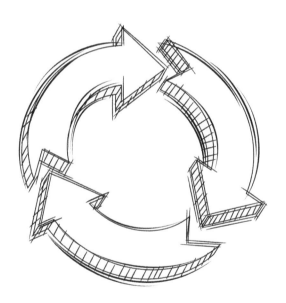

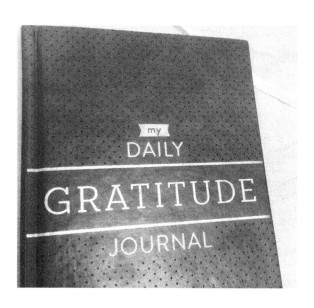

CHAPTER 13

The Paradox of Goals:

Habits, Routines, and Goal Setting

In preparing for battle I have always found that plans are useless,
but planning is indispensable.
– DWIGHT D. EISENHOWER

Lights, Camera…

And now for the REAL ACTION.

From breathwork, to blood work, to building stronger relationships, we've explored some of the most meaningful domains of our health. As we transition into the last act of this book, it's time we do just that—act.

In each of the preceding chapters, we've built a bit of action within each chapter and through the Action Items at the end of each chapter. Have you been following along and participating in those areas of action? If not, feel free to go back now and review some of those Action Items.

If you've already started taking some sort of new action in your health as you've read this book—kudos. Keep it up. And if you haven't taken much new action, but have done a lot of reflecting instead, that's great too. Now it's time to put it all together and build our Health Hacker Process and Game Plan.

Act 5 is devoted to empowering you to gather the major areas of your health together into one simple framework to implement on a daily and weekly basis. This is your chance to create your own unique plan of action.

I can't emphasize this enough: This is YOUR process and YOUR game plan. No one else's. One grave injustice in the health, wellness, and diet industries is the cookie-cutter, one-size-fits-all sort of approach to health optimization. This is the primary reason I wrote a book about self coaching and personal health empowerment rather than another how-to book.

This is about you and your own health. I'm simply highlighting ways you can approach your health and providing a mirror for you to see the results of your own self-coach, health-hacker approach.

Be Your Own Coach with a Health Hacker Approach

In this chapter, we now have a chance to set some goals and put our intention into action by exploring our habits, routines, and daily rituals.

Before we get into the paradox of goals, let's briefly reflect on where we stand and what we have learned about the concept of behavior change so far.

At the end of chapter 2, you were invited to take an inventory of your health. On a scale of 1 to 5, you rated both the Macro and Micro areas of your health. Go back and take another quick look at those ratings.

- Do you still agree with your ratings? Have any of those ratings changed throughout this book?
- Have you taken action or tried something new?
- Has your perspective on any area of health been impacted or changed?

Maybe you started journaling, went to bed a bit earlier, or started doing some breathwork first thing in the morning. Maybe you researched local functional medicine practitioners or started to remove certain foods from your diet. On a conscious or unconscious level, you're most likely in the process of considering or trying out a new behavior in your life.

That said, if you feel like you have more emotional processing to do before taking action, that's fine. It's actually encouraged. Just because you're taking action in your health for your future self doesn't mean you should forget about staying present your body and in your heart.

Remember, the key to health (and healing) is *integration*—in the moment and in the ever-changing phases and stages of life.

Five Stages of Change, Reviewed

As we discussed in chapter 6, the TTM of Behavior Change identifies five stages of change that most people experience:

1. Precontemplation (Not Ready): Not intending to change this behavior
2. Contemplation (Getting Ready): Intending to make this behavior change in the next six months
3. Preparation (Ready): Intending to make this behavior change in the next thirty days
4. Action: Have been engaging in the new behavior for less than six months
5. Maintenance: Have been engaging in the new behavior for more than six months

Can you relate to the idea that there are stages of change we go through in our lives?

At any given moment, we're at a different stage of change in our lives and, more specifically, our health. For example, you might be considering getting advanced blood work done to understand what's going on inside your body, but aren't quite sure where to start. Or you might be in a mode of transitioning one habit (such as shopping for healthier groceries at a farmers' market) from Preparation stage to Action stage. Or you may have a desire to have less stress—in work or in your relationships—which requires a courageous, honest, and intentional conversation with someone.

Wherever you are is fine. It's perfect, actually. The key is to put your "hat of awareness" on and be an observer of your own life. This model is not an end-all-be-all science, but a tool for transforming how you assess your interest in and readiness to explore a change in an area of your life.

As previously discussed, this model of behavior change was originally created for health practitioners to help patients move from one stage to the next in a sustainable way. This model may not have been created by or for us, but as health hackers, we can certainly benefit from this information to use in self coaching and buddy coaching.

Assessing our readiness to change is a handy tool for exploring our goals and getting ready to take action, but if we want to *build* our readiness to change and set sustainable goals fueled by intrinsic motivation, there are two powerful elements to consider.

Importance and Confidence

The behavior change process is just that—a process. It doesn't happen overnight. Understanding your readiness to try something new can bring a sense of peace and effortlessness to your self-coach approach. But, according to Rollnick, Mason, and Butler in their book, *Health Behavior Change: A Guide for Practitioners*, "If a change feels *important* to you, and you have the *confidence* to achieve it, you will feel more *ready* to have a go, and are more likely to succeed." As these authors point out, if we want to build our readiness to change, we must also create clarity about the **importance** of a goal and our **confidence** in our ability to carry that goal out.

- **Importance**—As we assess our readiness to change or try something new, it is critical that we assess how important a particular action or behavior is to us and our health. And what elements impact how important something is to us? Our values, as well as an understanding of what's possible if we do it and what's possible if we don't do it. So, as you explore a change in your health or a specific health goal, remember WHY it's important to you. This can fuel your motivation to change and define your reason for trying out a new healthy habit.

- **Confidence**—As we embark on the process of action, limiting beliefs can come up from time to time about our ability to succeed in a new behavior. Maybe it's new to us. Maybe we don't know how to cook, bake, work out, or find the right health care team. These thoughts or beliefs can result in low confidence. As you check in with yourself and your level of confidence in a particular healthy habit, guard against judging yourself or your experience. It's alright if you don't have the highest level of confidence yet. You don't have to be perfect. The key is to simply explore how you can build confidence in your approach.

Determining the importance of a habit or behavior and assessing our confidence level about making a change often go completely unnoticed. This can lead us to never take action in the first place or to make changes in a forceful, unsustainable way.

The simple questions become:

- How do we build the **confidence** necessary to achieve the outcomes we desire?
- How do we grow our awareness and understanding around the **importance** of learning and experimenting with new aspects of our health?

That's where intentional conversations through self coaching and buddy coaching enter the picture.

Conversation Flow Model and Self-Coaching Exercise

I first learned and experienced this Conversation Flow Model in the *The Clinical Health Coach Training* program. Let's put it into practice in this self-coaching exercise. The following steps are used by some health coaches to help influence sustainable behavior change with clients and patients:

1. Engaging
2. Focusing
3. Evoking Change Talk
4. Planning
5. Closing

To see the first three steps in action, I've provided a list of key questions to ask yourself. These are the exact questions I ask myself and my clients when exploring healthy habit behavior change:

1. Engaging

What's going well for you in your health?

In chapter 3, we discussed the value of *approving* of ourselves before we *improve* our health. As humans, it can be easy to focus on what we want to **fix, change, or improve.** The true art of health hacking comes into play when we can first acknowledge ourselves for the *good* we're doing in our lives and give ourselves a little self-love and acknowledgement before we transition into the areas of our health that may need some work.

2. Focusing

Have there been any new healthy habits you've tried in the past few weeks or months? What have you learned from these experiences?

This is a chance to reflect on recent life experiences and what we've learned about ourselves along the way.

If there are a few areas of your health you would consider exploring, what might those be? Why?

Because our total health picture can sometimes be overwhelming, this question allows us to consider multiple areas of our health—to start broad and then narrow it down to a few of the micro areas of our health to consider exploring.

3. Evoking Change Talk

Why is now a good time to try out those new habits or behaviors?

This is a chance to solidify why *now* is a good time to try out this new habit or behavior. This question helps create clarity about the importance of any goals we might set.

On a scale of 1 to 10, with 10 being the most important, how IMPORTANT is it for you to try this new behavior?

This is a chance for you to think about the importance of making this change, which may result in building the level of importance in your mind.

On a scale of 1 to 10, with 10 being the most confident, how CONFIDENT are you about moving forward with trying this new healthy habit or behavior?

This is a chance for you to get clear on your confidence level. Studies show if you're not a 7 or higher with respect to your confidence level, you may have a harder time following through with that habit.

Why did you give yourself the score you did? For example, if you rated your confidence level a 6, why not a 4?

This is a powerful question I often use as a health coach. It's a chance for you to provide reasons why you're confident about trying something new, which can result in even more confidence in yourself and your ability to make a change. For example, if you rated your confidence level in one area a 6, asking yourself key questions can actually build your confidence in this new habit or behavior, possibly bumping your rating to a 7 or 8.

Use the C.O.A.C.H. Approach

Through each of these exercises, remember to follow this simple acronym:

Choose This Moment…and Breathe
Observe Your Experience…and Feel
Assess Your Stress…and Heal
Communicate with Clarity…and Trust
Have Fun and Smile…You're Bound to Stay Awhile

I created the C.O.A.C.H. approach to provide you with a simple way to remember how to approach moments in life (as opposed to decisions about the future) that impact your health. In other words, it's not about planning, but about responding to what unfolds in your experience.

Now that we've gotten clear on how we can use the Conversation Flow Model and the C.O.A.C.H Approach to coach ourselves in our own health, let's transition into what this chapter is all about—a proper approach to goal setting.

The Paradox of Goals

In the behavior change world, we often refer to two types of goals: long-term, outcome-based goals and short-term, behavior-based goals.

After studying the leading-edge science of behavior change through various health coaching trainings, I've learned goal setting can seem like a paradox. Goals can be a great way of providing direction and guidance, but only focusing on long-term, outcome-based goals rather than short-term, behavior-based goals can leave us living in the future and not the present. Plus, if we don't reach our outcome goal, we may feel dejected or like a failure, which wouldn't be true!

It's our behaviors, our ability to live in the present, and our daily systems of habits and routines that can lead to reaching the goals and, ultimately, the feelings we desire. We can talk about change forever. But if we want to see real results, we must transition from talking the talk to walking the walk. Let us allow our actions and the ways we take care of ourselves to bring honor and meaning to this beautiful journey of life.

One of my favorite behavior change leaders is James Clear. In a blog post titled "Forget about Setting Goals. Focus on This Instead," Clear teaches people how to build better habits through "systems thinking," which focuses on engaging in specific behaviors or processes in pursuit of a goal. Clear highlights three reasons to focus on systems instead of goals:

- **Goals reduce happiness**
  Solution: Commit to a process, not a goal
- **Goals are strangely at odds with long-term progress**
  Solution: Release the need for immediate results
- **Goals suggest you can control things you have no control over**
  Solution: Build feedback loops

Can you relate to these reasons for shifting focus away from long-term goals? This concept is a great wake-up call for us to reflect on how we relate to goal setting, perhaps based on past experiences or current interests. But you don't have to forget about setting goals altogether. Goals aren't useless. As Clear reiterates in his article, "I've found that goals are good for planning your progress and systems are good for actually making progress." If you like the idea of creating goals to hold you accountable in your health, great. Go for it! Just make sure you are mindful of how you approach change and goal setting in general.

As a health coach, I'm not going to tell you *not* to set goals if you want to set goals. But I *am* going to help you focus on the short-term, behavior-based goals or systems that lead and propel you toward the outcomes you desire.

S.M.A.R.T. Goals

The following exercise will explain what a S.M.A.R.T. goal is and the difference between Micro and Macro S.M.A.R.T. goals.

What is a **S.M.A.R.T.** goal?

- **Specific**–What do I want to accomplish? What is the purpose or benefit of accomplishing the goal?
- **Measurable**–Establish solid criteria for measuring progress toward the achievement of each goal you set.
- **Attainable**–Identify your most important goals. Program your thoughts, habits, environment, and actions toward these goals.
- **Realistic**–You are the only one who can decide how ambitious your goal should be. But be sure that every goal represents substantial progress. Remember, it's about progress, not perfection.
- **Time-bound**–All goals should have a time constraint. Without this element, there is no sense of urgency. If you want to lose twenty pounds, how soon do you want to lose it? "Someday" won't work. But if you anchor it within a timeframe (e.g., by April 15, 2017), you've trained your unconscious mind to begin working on the goal.

There are two different types of S.M.A.R.T. Goals: Micro Goals and Macro Goals.

Micro S.M.A.R.T. Goals:
- **Short-term (daily, weekly) behavior-based goals** that involve executing a plan, which helps big (macro) goals happen.

- Micro S.M.A.R.T. Goal Example:
  - Replace pop/soda with a healthy alternative (e.g., spring water with sea salt and lemon, sparkling water with lime or Zevia) that mimics soda in its taste, but has less sugar and artificial sweeteners that can negatively impact your health.
  - Commitment: I will buy a case of sparkling mineral water when I go to the grocery store this Saturday.
- Does it meet all of the criteria of a S.M.A.R.T. goal? I think it does!

Macro S.M.A.R.T. Goals:

- **Long term, outcome-based goals** made possible by following micro or behavior-based goals.
  - Macro S.M.A.R.T. Goal Example:
- I will lose ten pounds of fat and gain five pounds of muscle by April 15, 2018.
- Does it meet all of the criteria of a S.M.A.R.T. goal? Yes.

As we discussed in Act 4, there are several other areas of our health (e.g., stress levels, micronutrient deficiencies, annual lab work) to consider measuring if we want to make a larger impact on both our short-term and long-term health future.

Knowing the difference between these two types of goals and the importance of focusing on behavior based goals can help build a healthier relationship with goal setting in general. But there are other fundamental philosophical approaches that can help as well.

The Experimental Mindset

Lately, I've enjoyed viewing my new behaviors and health habits as experiments. This strategy has brought a lot of ease to how I approach my health. Integrating principles from the scientific method can lead to an experimental mindset—to have an intention of what you're testing with a hypothesis in mind—but less attachment to the outcome and more focus on the process.

What if we looked at our habits and health behaviors as an experiment?

Could this be one of the core fundamentals for creating sustainable behavior change?

That's what Tony Stubblebine, Chief Coach at Coach.Me, believes. In an interview for this book, Coach Tony indicated two key principles that separate the "successful" from the "unsuccessful" as it relates to creating healthy habits: Experimentation and Momentum.

- **Experimentation**–Making changes to better our lives requires desire and motivation, but it also takes action. According to Coach Tony, "When most try to change a habit, it's all or nothing. When in all actuality they need to put together a system to find out the thing that works for them. That's a mindset shift toward experimentation and trial and error. And away from the all-or-nothing approach." The sort of shift Coach Tony is advocating for leads to a deeper level of ease with less attachment to the outcome.

- **Momentum**–As we start to see small amounts of success in how we feel and even our ability to complete certain tasks or behaviors, we start to progress and experience momentum. "Momentum is a second area to focus on," Coach Tony explains. "Once you start having a number of victories, your mindset changes to think you can have more." I completely agree.

What if instead of focusing 100 percent on being successful with a goal, we could enjoy the journey a bit more and learn a thing or two along the way? Adopting an experimental mindset can be our greatest tool as health hackers. Improving health and addressing behavior change is not a succeed or fail proposition—unless you make it that. If you approach it like an experiment you become much more patient with yourself and the outcome becomes less personal. You are simply a scientist testing the subject of an experiment, and the focus can shift to what you learn about yourself through the process. The process is where the growth occurs, not necessarily in reaching a quantitative metric at the end of a specified time period.

And, as Coach Tony points out, any successes that are observed thanks to this mindset can help create the momentum needed to believe you will experience more success.

As long as we focus on the intention of our actions and see them as an experiment, goals can be great. **The key is to learn throughout the process and focus on short-term habits, not long-term goals.**

Healthy Habit Feedback Loops

There is a great opportunity for us to put this experimental mindset into action as we build an important practice: Healthy Habit Feedback Loops.

What's a feedback loop, exactly?

Feedback loops, traditionally discussed in relation to economics, machinery, or nature, refer to outputs informing inputs.

As you may recall, behavior change expert James Clear advocates for a systems approach to building better habits. As Clear explains, "Feedback loops are important for building good systems because they allow you to keep track of many different pieces without feeling the pressure to predict what is going to happen with everything."

Feedback loops also relate to our health and our ability to improve and grow.

You've probably started connecting the dots between decisions about your health, and how those decisions relate to how you feel and operate as a high-performing human:

- If I eat sugar or drink too much caffeine or alcohol, I feel like crap.
- If I eat well, move my body, and get quality rest, I feel pretty good.

In the behavior change world, we call these mechanisms **Feedback Loops** of cause and effect: behavior X (input) produces result Y (output), and that result (output) is used to adjust future behavior (input).

There are two types of feedback loops:

- **Reinforcing Feedback Loops**–These feedback loops are used to moderate "good" habits. For example, if you feel good after a workout, yoga, or movement session and that positive feeling leads you to want to do it again the next day, you have created a reinforcing feedback loop.
- **Balancing Feedback Loops**–These feedback loops are used to moderate "bad" habits. For example, a flashing sign on the side of the road displaying your current driving speed next to the actual speed limit in an attempt at creating a balancing feedback loop to prevent speeding.

Build Your Own Feedback Loops

Here are some examples of feedback loops you can deploy in your own health:

1. Measure blood work before and after a nutrition, supplement, or other lifestyle change, and then use that information to inform future health behaviors.
2. Engage in conscious conversations with friends and family to ask for feedback about their experience of you in relationship to them, and then use that information to consider making a change in your behavior.
3. Use a wearable (like the Oura Ring, discussed in chapter 14) to track your sleep, movement, or nutrition, and then make adjustments to these areas of health based on the data you collect.
4. Measure your heart rate and blood pressure before and after you spend time in nature to see if or how it changes.

Within these feedback loops and our overall approach to behavior change, it's also important to understand the difference between habits and routines.

Habits vs. Routines

In my opinion, the key to a healthy lifestyle is to create a balance between healthy habits and healthy routines. And, perhaps more importantly, to understand how healthy routines can turn into healthy habits.

So what is the difference between habits and routines, exactly?

- **Habits** are behaviors done with little or no conscious thought and require less mental and emotional energy—they are carried out as though on autopilot.
- **Routines** are patterns you consciously create in your life with a bit more thought, effort, and energy.

Taking a good look at our habits and routines will help us stay focused on creating healthy habits that matter. And if we really want to take our health hacking game to another level, I suggest we experiment with something even more powerful—habit stacking.

The Health Hacker Habit Stacker

As we've discussed in the past, when it comes to creating healthy habits, **we're better off focusing our energies on creating new habits instead of simply breaking bad ones.** Don't get me wrong, having the goal and interest to break a perceived bad habit is great. But to truly see the habit go away for good, we need to replace it with something else.

What if instead of just focusing on one new habit at a time, we focused on one state at a time—how we want to think, feel, and operate in any given moment?

For example, let's say you want to avoid the habit of watching television before bed, or spending less time with technology late at night because you want to see how it might be impacting your sleep.

With the underlying goal of the experiment being higher quality of sleep, there are a lot of tactics you could try.

You could replace your habit of watching television or being on your computer, tablet, or phone with a new habit, perhaps reading a book. But there's a problem—there still may be a decent level of temptation to use your phone or computer. You've only tried to replace your habit of late night technology use with one habit (reading a book).

Now let's say, instead of just focusing on one new habit to replace the bad habit, you were to focus on multiple habits—specific habits and behaviors that, when put together, could help support your overall goal of deepening your state of rest and relaxation before bed.

That's what is referred to as habit stacking.

Habit stacking is the process of combining certain small behaviors together within a short period of time to help the brain and body create a desired state.

You can apply this habit stacking process to anything, really. But for the purposes of this book and my work in health hacking, I like to help people use this process with health-hacker habits.

I call it the **Health Hacker Habit Stacker.**

What if, instead of just reading to replace your technology use, you also chose to brew a pot of lavender tea, take a magnesium supplement, or hop into a warm Epsom salt bath with some relaxing music playing in the background before changing into your pajamas?

With any process, following the right steps becomes very important if you want to achieve desired results. That's why I created a three-step process to help you experiment with the Health Hacker Habit Stacker in your daily life.

Note: This is designed to be applied and followed during certain time periods of your day. Not just as a theoretical concept. So take action, my friends!

Step 1–Get Clear on What You Want

The first step is to figure out what you want in the moment. What is the set and setting? And what is the desired state do you want to create?

You can start rushing to new routines and habits, but until you decide what state you want to create, you won't have your compass in check to guide you through the process.

Important Note: Don't limit yourself. You can desire multiple states at once, not just one. For example, you can desire peace and focus at the same time. Or you can desire relaxation and creativity at the same time.

Step 2–Make a List and Make a Move

After you choose the state you want to create, make a list of all the different behaviors or activities that could help you create that state.

Let's use the rest and relaxation before bed example again here.

If you want to break the habit of being on technology before bed, or at least test the impact that changing this habit could have, what are all the activities and behaviors that could possibly help support you in this quest of getting better sleep? Here are some ideas:

- Read a book
- Change into your pajamas
- Take a walk outside
- Do some stretching
- Take specific supplement, like magnesium or CBD
- Brew a pot of lavender tea or make a Reishi mushroom drink
- Take a warm Epsom salt bath
- Use essential oils associated with relaxation (Lavender, Chamomile, etc.)
- Do breathwork that promotes relaxation
- Listen to relaxing music
- Turn off all the lights in the room or house and use candles instead

Choose as many or as few of these ideas as you want. If these are all new to you, I would suggest only starting with a few. The fewer you start with, the easier it is to test the incremental impact.

Step 3–Notice and Reflect

After you choose to start trying out some of these new activities or behaviors, the last important step is to **notice** how you feel and **reflect** on the experience.

- What did you notice?
- What did you experience?
- How did you feel?
- What did you learn?

You can easily repeat this simple, three-step process in the same area of your life, or ride the momentum of success in one area of your life by following these steps in a different area of your life. Just make sure you're mindful of not making too many changes in your lifestyle all at once, and remember, it is the process of planning, rather than the specific plan, that will allow us to see the results that living a more intentional, healthy lifestyle can provide.

By following the steps outlined in this chapter, we are well on our way to becoming our own health coach. Whether it's mental focus, physical energy, or more rest and relaxation, we have the ability to create the states we desire. All it takes is a bit of courage and intentional self-experimentation.

Summary:

- If you build the importance and confidence in your ability to change a behavior, you are more likely to succeed.
- Avoid the all-or-nothing approach to habit change. Instead, focus on the process itself and celebrate your incremental successes. This will help you shift your mindset toward experimentation and trial and error, so you can reflect on and learn from your experience.
- Focusing on the intention of our actions and viewing **goals as an experiment** can be great. The key is to learn throughout the process and focus on short-term habits, not long-term goals.
- Try out habit stacking with the **Health Hacker Habit Stacker** three-step process: Get Clear on What You Want, Make a List and Make a Move, Notice and Reflect.
- Consider using the **C.O.A.C.H. Approach** acronym, to remember how to approach moments in life (as opposed to decisions about the future) that impact your health. In other words, it's not all about planning, but about responding to what unfolds in your experience.

Choose This Moment
Observe Your Experience
Assess Your Stress
Communicate with Clarity
Have Fun and Smile

Action Items:

1. Go through the Conversation Flow Model and Self-Coaching Exercise again.

   • What is going on in your health? What is going well? What is not going well?

   • Is there anything in particular you're interested in improving?

   • Make a list of all the potential areas of your health you might consider changing.

   • Why would now be a good time to try out a new behavior or habit?

2. Review the five stages of change and assess the level of importance and confidence you have in each of those areas. Remember to ask yourself why you gave yourself the score you did—think of reasons that you're confident about trying something new.

3. Choose a habit or behavior to focus on and complete the following S.M.A.R.T. goal-setting exercise:

   • What are a few of your Macro (outcome-based) S.M.A.R.T. Goals?

   • What are the Micro (behavior-based) elements of each of these S.M.A.R.T. Goals?

4. Identify the steps in the Healthy Habit Loop for one of your behavior-based Micro goals above.

   • **Measure and Document**. Establish criteria for measuring progress and how you could best document that progress.

   • **Analyze.** After trying out the new behavior or habit, reflect on how you feel about what happened. What did you learn? What seemed interesting or relevant to you?

   • **Correct.** Respond with a course correction, like a change in mindset, environment, or conditions.

   • **Repeat.** Repeat the same activity in a different way, and the feedback loop continues.

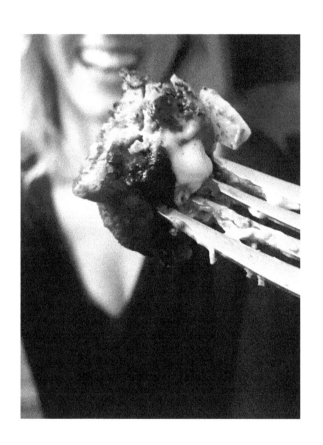

CHAPTER 14

Your Daily Routine:

Nutrition, Movement, and Sleep 101

The doctor of the future will no longer treat the human frame with drugs, but rather will cure and prevent disease with nutrition.
— THOMAS EDISON

We are entering the homestretch of this book. We've explored top strategies and principles for communicating with and relating to ourselves and others. We've learned about the role of feedback loops in our health, explored the difference between habits and routines, and completed both a self-coaching and habit-stacking exercise to set proper goals and integrate behavior change into our lives.

Now that we have a better idea of the habits we want to keep, create, or change, as well as the routines we need to help us get there, let's start putting them into action.

As a clinical health coach, the conversations I have with my clients, friends, and family can go in many different directions. But one of the most important things I've learned is to support people by helping them focus on three fundamental areas of health—Movement, Sleep, and Nutrition.

Let's explore how we currently relate to these fundamental areas of health and how we're all called to evolve our approach to building healthy habits that matter.

The truth is, we all have an intrinsic hunger and biological instinct to adapt and survive. But our calling as modern-day, health-conscious consumers is not just to adapt and survive, but to elevate and thrive. Other than air, water, plant life, and human connection, what else is most fundamental for human life? **The food we put inside our bodies.**

Nutrition 101

What is nutrition? Technically, it's anything you put inside your body that has nutrients. But not all food is equally nutritious. In other words, all food can be placed on a spectrum of low nutrition to high nutrition. There is a stark difference between eating food to survive and consuming food to thrive, so an essential commitment as health hackers is to use a lens of nutrition to explore what we eat and drink.

What are some things you already KNOW about nutrition?

Think about that for a moment. One of the first things I learned about nutrition was that there are three types of macronutrients—proteins, fats, and carbohydrates. But not all calories are created equal. On a cellular level, we are made up of a wide array of essential amino acids (proteins) and essential fatty acids (fats). We don't have essential carbohydrate acids in our body. You may have heard the general idea that carbs are not good for you. Technically, our cells require protein and fat more than carbs. But the modern-day, processed-food generation in which we're living means we're battling against dozens of companies and hundreds of brands that aim to dominate our taste buds.

Over the past five years, I've learned a lot about nutrition, and I'm still learning. I've had nutrition education in a few different health education and coach training curriculums, specifically *Healthy for Life University* and the *YMCA Health Coach Certification*. But most of what I've learned about nutrition was learned through self-study and self-experimentation. I've learned there is more to nutrition than science; rather, we can take an artful approach with respect to our food.

Now, not everyone reading this book may be as passionate about health and nutrition as I am. But you can still align your goals and motivations with learning more about one of the very things that allows you stay alive, prevent disease, and truly thrive.

You don't have to be a nutritionist or dietitian to learn about nutrition. You just need to find a strong enough interest and motivation to learn and experiment.

The primary reason I became enthralled with the power of food and nutrition for optimal health and performance was for myself—how I think, feel, and operate as a human.

While living in Miami, I read a book called *Grain Brain: The Surprising Truth about Wheat, Carbs, and Sugar—Your Brain's Silent Killers*. Dr. David Perlmutter writes about the impact of nutrition on the brain; specifically, how diets filled with sugar, grains, and processed carbohydrates are correlated with a higher risk of neurodegenerative diseases like Alzheimer's and dementia. That's when I started waking up to importance of healthy fat, stumbled upon the Bulletproof Diet, and decided to make some changes in my overall approach to eating.

Over the past two years, I've experimented with a high-fat (60 to 80 percent of total calories) ketogenic diet. This way of eating requires choosing to find and prepare specific kinds of food, not just eating it.

The ketogenic diet has grown in popularity over the past few years. Perhaps you've heard of it. But what is it really about and how does it work? One of the main intentions behind a ketogenic diet is to shift how your metabolism uses food as fuel. Specifically, the "keto" way of eating involves eating a high-fat, low-carb diet. Over time, you'll start to notice you receive most of your energy from healthy fat sources and are naturally able to reduce your use of carbohydrates and sugars for energy. In essence, you're shifting your metabolism from being carb adapted to fat adapted. And in my experience—both personally in my diet and professionally working with clients—this shift can work wonders for overall health, energy, as well as physical and mental performance. But it's important to note this shift can take six to eight weeks, give or take a few weeks, depending on your current level of health, your approach, and also your gender. (Women don't always do as well following a strict ketogenic diet due to its impact on hormones, but it still may be worth experimenting.)

If you're interested in trying it out for yourself, but want a bit more direction, I suggest you take a look at *Grain Brain* by Dr. David Perlmutter or *The Bulletproof Diet* by Dave Asprey. You can also check out Asprey's free Bulletproof Diet Roadmap Infographic online. It's a great starting point for approaching the idea of experimenting with a higher fat, lower carbohydrate diet.

It's important to note that the ketogenic diet is not for everyone. It impacts the body differently for everyone, and can even affect your level of hydration. If you do give it a try, make sure you are consuming more high-quality sea salt than you did before you made this change to your diet. As you read earlier, I paid a visit to the ER for low sodium. While there were several factors related to this visit, I believe my approach to this high-fat, low-carb diet was a contributing factor. Put simply, I wasn't eating enough salt and had also pulled some hydrating foods out of my diet. It's also important to get and reference blood work and genetics when considering a major change in your way of eating.

Regardless of which diet you follow, it's important to realize what you eat impacts everything—how you think, how you feel, and how you function as a human being. As such, we need to understand not just what foods to eat, but also what foods to avoid eating.

During the past two decades, there has been a huge increase in rates of obesity among adults and children. There are several reasons for this; one of which, the types of food people eat. Another, the amount of chemicals that make up today's food flavor profiles.

Today we have 2,200 flavor chemicals meant to mimic naturally occurring foods on the market—an increase of 1,500 flavor chemicals over the past fifty years! In a *Medical Daily* article titled "The Food Industry Has Changed How Our Taste Buds Work," Samantha Olson highlights how this has impacted our current state of health and nutrition: "A once simple system of nutritional nourishment has been toyed with by a complex, chemically-altered language that our bodies are now struggling to communicate with."

In this article, Olson highlights another book that dives deep into this topic—*The Dorito Effect: The Surprising Truth About Food and Flavor*. As author and food journalist Mark Schatzker explains, "We could live in a world where food tastes very good and the people who eat it are not fat." In other words, we could have an entirely different experience of food and, in turn, lower rates of obesity. Let's look to the future of food and nutrition. Is it up to us as consumers to become, as some health hackers would say, "bulletproof," by avoid harmful foods and drinks? Well, yes, focusing on what we can do on our own is wildly important. But the right organizations in positions of power and several positive movements are starting to change the world of nutrition to support our efforts.

In fall 2016, the World Health Organization (WHO) published the report *Fiscal Policies for Diet and Prevention of Noncommunicable Diseases* that announced several proposed policy recommendations for improving nutrition, including a 20 percent tax on sugary drinks. Regardless of how you feel about laws like a sugar tax, this goes to show how our world is starting to wake up to the seriousness of our health situation.

> But once we, as individuals, realize how sugar is bad for us, how do we move forward? How can we eat less sugar so it doesn't wreak havoc on our health?

In the book *The Sugar Impact Diet*, author and celebrity nutrition expert JJ Virgin offers up a different approach for people to consider that will help them be more successful while trying to reduce their sugar intake. Virgin outlines three different cycles—Taper, Transition, and Transform—intended to be followed sequentially as individuals wean themselves off sugar.

During our interview, Virgin explained how she helps people lose fat and ditch sugar cravings using the concept of Tapering:

> If you go cold turkey on sugar, you will fail. First, you need to start tapering—lowering your sugar intake gradually over a week or two. Go from high sugar impact foods, like a white potato, to medium sugar impact foods, like a sweet potato.

Transformation doesn't happen overnight, and neither do the processes that lead to transformation. If you're someone who struggles with sugar or carbs and wants to find a way to make more progress in getting off these foods and drinks, I highly suggest you check out one of Virgin's many books or cookbooks (specifically, *The Sugar Impact Diet*), and take her Sugar Impact Quiz online to see how much of an impact sugar is having on your life.

So, we know sugar is bad for us, and now we have some resources to help us approach eating less of it, but how do we put it all together? What are some of the top principles for us to focus on when it comes to nutrition?

People often ask about how I eat or what diet I follow. The best way to describe how I eat is to list the main ways I've changed my approach to nutrition over the past seven years. Perhaps these principles of eating will help you in your journey as well.

Ten Fundamental Ways I've Evolved My Eating Habits

1. Eat for performance and pleasure
2. Breathe before and during meals
3. Eat slowly and stop eating at 80 percent full
4. Eat based on intuition
5. Daily and weekly fasting
6. Eat with my blood work in mind
7. Cut out processed foods and eat whole foods in their original state
8. Eat seasonally and locally
9. Cut out all grain-fed, non-pastured meat and replace with local, organic, grass-fed (and grass-finished) pastured meat or wild-caught fish
10. Eat more healthy fat and fewer inflammatory, high glycemic-based foods

Eat for performance and pleasure. It's OK to view food as fuel, because that's what it is. And quality fuel will give you quality energy. It's also important to eat quality food for enjoyment and pleasure. Just because you want to eat healthy doesn't mean you have to lose the enjoyment of creating and eating food. If you do the research and experiment with new ways to cook healthier food with great ingredients, you will quickly realize how easy it can be to make healthy food taste great!

Breathe before and during meals. Your brain lags behind your stomach in realizing that you are full. So to prevent overeating, it's important to slow down your pace of eating by taking time to breath. This time spent breathing will allow you to be more aware of what your body needs and how full it feels.

Eat slowly and stop eating at 80 percent full. As previously mentioned, your brain lags behind your stomach. So when you stop eating at 80 percent full and wait about ten to fifteen minutes, your food can continue digesting to the point that your brain receives a signal that you are now, in fact, full. If you're still hungry, have a little bit more to eat; If you're not still hungry, don't.

To see the benefit of this practice, take a moment right now to reflect on how full you usually feel after a meal. If you feel like you ever become uncomfortably full, it may be wise to consider doing an experiment:

1. Slow down when you eat, pausing and breathing between each bite.
2. Set an intention to pause toward the end of your meal, waiting ten to fifteen minutes to see how you feel.
3. If you're still hungry, eat a little bit more, repeating the steps above. If you are no longer hungry, stop eating.

Slow down, breathe, and set your intention to be mindful of your level of fullness. These steps may seem simple, but it is important to view them as an experiment and not as a success or failure. Afterward, reflect on what you learned from the meal, just as you would if you were doing a science experiment.

Eat based on intuition. This one is hard to describe. But let me first say eating based on intuition is not simply eating what you crave. Rather, you must tap into what your body *needs* to feel better. So ask yourself what your body desires and listen.

Daily and weekly fasting. There are more and more studies coming out every year about the benefits of short-term, intermittent fasting. If done correctly and for the right reasons, fasting can have several health benefits, including, but not limited to, detoxification, reduced inflammation, improved cardiovascular health, decreased likelihood of obesity, and relief from pain-inducing conditions like arthritis. Fasting can also help the body heal and burn fat faster, as it stimulates the release of growth hormone. I highly recommend experimenting with intermittent fasting, such as a daily twelve- to sixteen-hour fast (sleeping counts!) or a twenty-four-hour fast once or twice a week. **Always consult your doctor first, especially if you have any other health or medical conditions.**

Eat with my blood work in mind. We covered this a bit earlier, but eating based on what's going on inside your body—your heart, hormones, thyroid, gut, and micronutrient levels—can make a big difference in avoiding sickness and staying healthy. For example, if your blood work shows certain markers are elevated, nutrition usually plays a primary role in adjusting these levels.

Cut out overly processed foods and eat whole foods in their original state as much as possible. Eating healthy isn't just about eating the right foods, but about avoiding the wrong ones. When you replace overly processed foods with foods that contain minimal ingredients (usually in their whole state), your health and energy will change for the better. Plus, over time, you can re-train your taste buds to actually enjoy whole food!

Eat seasonally and locally. I'm not perfect at this, but it is my intention to eat as seasonally and locally as possible. There is a reason certain foods grow better at certain times of the year—because we are meant to consume different foods! Eating locally is important if you want to support your local farmer, but it can also help ensure you're eating the freshest food possible with minimal transportation and storage time.

Cut out all grain-fed, non-pastured meat and replace with local, organic, grass-fed (and grass-finished) pastured meat or wild-caught fish. Avoid any meats with nitrates and growth hormones. One of the best ways to source high-quality meat is through your local farmers' market. But make sure you do your research and ask your farmers good questions! Understanding where animals come from, what they eat, and how they're treated is very important to the nutrition of the food and to our entire ecosystem.

Eat more healthy fat and less inflammatory, high-glycemic foods. For the past several decades, fat has been demonized as unhealthy for the body. We think of fat on the body as bad, and so we look at fat, the nutrient, as bad too. But it's not. In fact, consuming enough calories from fat is essential for our cells. The key is to focus on eating healthy fats (from foods like avocados, nuts, seeds, eggs, coconuts, and well-sourced animal proteins), and avoiding unhealthy fats (like most vegetable oils and grain-fed dairy) and too much sugar or high-glycemic carbohydrates. Because, according to recent research, diets filled with high-glycemic carbohydrates and unhealthy fats tend to create the inflammation in the body that leads to disease.

Bonus Health Hacker Tip: Innovate your desserts with less sugar and more healthy fat.

While writing this book, my girlfriend Amanda helped me evolve how I approach eating dessert. I didn't want eating dessert to be an activity in which I invited guilt. Instead, I've learned to focus on making my desserts different in the first place—without harmful ingredients and high amounts of sugar—so they not only taste great, but nourish and empower my brain and body as well.

While this isn't a cookbook, I'll still leave you with one of my favorite dessert recipes. Amanda shared this "Fat Bomb" recipe with me when we were living in Venice, California, and now I recommend it to everyone who wants to enjoy guilt-free and health-ful dessert. It's the best tasting and healthiest dessert I've ever had. Try it for yourself—your brain, body, and taste buds will thank you. Enjoy!

Fat Bombs
Ingredients:

2–3 tablespoons raw cacao

3–4 tablespoons of coconut oil

2 tablespoons MCT oil

4 tablespoons of sunflower seed butter (I recommend Sun Butter brand—the best sugar-free sunflower seed butter on the planet. But if you can tolerate nuts, you can also use any sugar-free nut butter of your choice.)

1 teaspoon vanilla extract

1 tablespoon local, raw honey or a few drops of liquid stevia

A dash of sea salt

A few handfuls of shredded coconut

Directions:

1. Place all ingredients, except the shredded coconut, into a pot on the stove.
2. Stir on medium heat, mixing until ingredients are incorporated and melted.
3. Once melted into a liquid, mix in shredded coconut.
4. Pour the liquid chocolate creation into an ice cube tray (or chocolate/candy mold).
5. Place the ice cube tray in your freezer, and allow to sit for at least one to two hours (and up to overnight) depending on your freezer. Don't consume until fully frozen.
6. You can store these nearly sugar free, high-fat, superfood Fat Bombs in the freezer to enjoy throughout your week.

    Note: I recommend trying only one Fat Bomb (that fits in one ice cube hole) to start. The fat content in this recipe is high, and depending on your stomach and how it handles high-fat foods (specifically MCT oil), you may experience disaster pants (i.e., intestinal discomfort).

    When preparing dessert, or any food for that matter, consider using a simple acronym to help you keep the process healthy, simple, and fun: **K**ey **I**ngredients, **S**imple **S**teps (KISS).

In closing our section on nutrition, I'll leave you with a powerful quote and metaphor from JJ Virgin: "Your body isn't a bank account. It's a chemistry lab. And food is the most powerful information you can give your body."

Allow this idea to stick with you. Keep listening to and learning about how your body responds to different foods. You'll be much better off because of it.

Supplements and Nootropics 101

Now that we've covered some fundamental hacks we can make to our food-based nutrition approach, let's take a look at how we can experiment with optimizing the supplement-based nutrients we consume to promote the states we want to create.

When it comes to supplements, I'm pretty intentional about what I put in my body. But as a health coach, entrepreneur, and a self-experimenting health hacker, if the research checks out, I'm always interested in trying something new to elevate my state of health and focus, as well as my mental and physical performance.

First, I want to be clear in saying I suggest people focus on optimizing their relationship with food before getting into supplements.

Second, as discussed in chapter 11, I suggest you approach supplements based on what's actually going on inside your body through blood work and genetics. That means working with your physician and health care team to determine what, if any, deficiencies and food allergies or sensitivities you may have. As we learned earlier from SpectraCell nutrition consultant Kirstin Keilty, nutrition is a concert—not a solo. Adding a particular supplement into our lifestyle doesn't just impact us in the one way we want it to; rather, depending on the supplement, other key vitamins and micronutrients are impacted in some way. That's why it's suggested that supplement plans be customized around individuals' blood work and genetics, involving someone trained in that field (e.g., a holistic nutritionist or naturopathic doctor).

Once you have addressed these two areas, you can develop a bit more freedom in your daily supplement approach to create specific states—how you want to think, feel, and perform—throughout your days.

We've talked a bit about supplements in the context of stress already, but what are some ways we can use supplements to bring more energy, clarity, and mental focus to our day? That's where nootropics come in.

What are nootropics?

Nootropics are supplements specifically designed to help enhance cognitive function in some way—boosting our real-time ability to focus, manage our memory, and activate a more creative state of being.

Sometimes called "smart drugs," nootropics are known for increasing communication between neurons and helping to balance neurotransmitter levels to promote powerful brain health. Often the benefits of nootropics are the result of combining certain ingredients together that on their own have one effect, but when taken together, amplify or enhance that effect. In fact, you may have tried a nootropic-like substance before without even realizing it.

Take caffeine, for example. Technically, caffeine by itself can act like a nootropic by increasing mental or physical energy. Furthermore, by combining caffeine and green tea (more specifically, L-theanine, a naturally occurring ingredient found in green tea), you can get a lift from the caffeine and a sense of calm from L-theanine.

Let's take a look at some of the leading health, nutrition, and human performance startups taking this concept to a whole new level.

Enter Neurohacker Collective

The world of nootropics and supplements is filled with many clickbait capitalists trying to make a quick buck. So many of these companies are claiming to heal and cure a lot of conditions. What's more, most of the products out there are of very poor quality. But that doesn't mean all companies and formulations are bad.

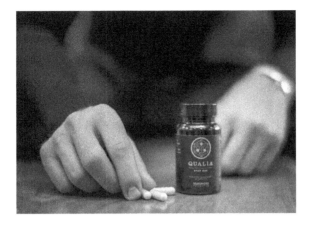

A few years ago, during my vagabonding adventures through San Diego, I learned about a new, up-and-coming neurotechnology company called Neurohacker Collective. Based out of Encinitas, California, Neurohacker has created a powerful nootropic stack supplement called Qualia. At first I was a bit hesitant, but after getting to know their team and learning more about the company and the science of their supplements, I became intrigued by their approach.

The research behind their first product, Qualia, is remarkable. Rooted in clean, whole-systems complexity science, these guys are taking the nootropics industry to a whole level. Not only does Qualia provide short term benefits of more energy and focus, but also long term benefits of new neuron and synapse development as well as increased mitochondrial ATP. Plus, they don't hide their formulation; instead, they talk openly on their website and in their podcasts about the sourcing, amount, and purpose of each of the forty-two ingredients in Qualia.

Before I recommend a supplement these days, the human guinea pig in me wants to learn more about the research and try the product myself. So that's what I did. After taking Qualia on and off for ten months, I've noticed a subtle, calm sense of focus coupled with a new level of mind-body alertness like I've never experienced before. Qualia allows the light bulb in the brain to be turned on to another level, while still remaining somewhat peaceful in my body. Cognitive function is dialed in, but there aren't many physical jitters or crashes. I truly feel like I am thinking, feeling, and performing at my best when I take it.

So if you're looking for a healthier and more sustainable way to stay focused, think clearly, and feel and perform at your best, Qualia just might be worth looking into. Visit http://Neurohacker.com to learn more.

What are the downsides of nootropics?

Are nootropics addictive? Are the ingredients harmful? Are there any side effects? Hollywood movies and television shows provide us with plenty of fictional examples of these sorts of magic smart-drug pills. So it's not surprising that a lot of people may be turned off when they hear "brain-boosting smart drugs," perhaps wondering about the potential downsides of taking such pills.

Nootropics are not intended to be an everyday essential supplement. As with caffeine, there could be a risk of developing a dependency (i.e., changing the body's natural processes to require the variable to function or to experience withdrawal when discontinued) on a tolerance (i.e., create a diminished response) to the ingredients in nootropics.

This is where the concept of cycling comes into play.

Embrace Cycling

What is cycling? The principle of cycling suggests you partake in a specific nutrition or supplement habit for a period of time, then stop the habit temporarily. Cycling on and off specific types of vitamins, minerals, and other ingredients, allows our brains, bodies, and entire biochemical processes to take a break from certain variables so as not to build up a dependency or tolerance to those variables.

In fact, Neurohacker suggests people cycle on and off Qualia as well—five days on, two days off, plus one full week off per month. In other words, cycling is built into the fabric of Qualia. For me, it feels like a great tool to be able to take whenever I desire a bit more energy, focus, and creativity to get through important work projects—taking it about two to four times per week.

In the interest of full disclosure, Qualia is not for everyone. Per their website, "this product contains chemicals that should not be taken by people on MAO inhibitors, SSRIs, or any other psychiatric medicines…people with psychiatric or neurologic disorders, high blood pressure, heart conditions, endocrine disorders, cancer, or people on immunosuppressive therapy…pregnant or nursing mothers, or children under 18." Additionally, if you are sensitive to caffeine, you may want to avoid Qualia, or at least start with a microdose (smaller than the suggested dose). If you already consume a lot of caffeine (e.g., coffee or tea), you may want to consider cutting back on other sources before you try a product like Qualia.

Their suggested serving size is three Step One capsules on an empty stomach (usually first thing in the morning) and six (caffeine-free) Step Two capsules later in the day with food. This amounts to roughly 100 mg of caffeine (33mg per capsule)—about the same amount found in a twelve-ounce cup of coffee. I usually suggest starting with 1–2 capsules, and then work up from there as necessary. That's how I use it. But it requires a case-by-case, customized approach for everyone.

The name of their supplement, Qualia, speaks to what we're all aiming for in this world—optimizing the quality of our human experience. Neurohacker is not just another supplement or nootropic company, but one of the leaders in the neurohacking and health optimization movement. Focused on curating the most meaningful technology in the neuro-tech space, Neurohacker is a purpose-driven collective that partners with other organizations doing meaningful work to upgrade our civilization. I had a chance to interview co-founder and head of Research & Development, Daniel Schmachtenberger, about their organization, the health care system, and how we "do" civilization in general. According to Schmachtenberger,

We affect and are affected by our environment. If there are more toxins in the environment than are in our bodies, they will diffuse in until they are equal. This is how osmosis works. If the nutrients aren't in the soil due to poor agricultural practices, they won't be in our bodies. Our health and the health of our world are inseparable topics. The future of medicine has to involve the future of agriculture, pollution, education…everything that affects individual well-being.

It's our responsibility as health hackers to do our own research and experiment with what we feel called to try. In addition to Neurohacker Collective, there are several other nootropic and supplement companies I would suggest looking into. Here are some of my other favorite companies and products:

- **Natural Stacks**
  - ○ MagTech Magnesium supplement
  - ○ Branched Chain Amino Acids (BCAAs)
- **EAD Labs** (Creator of BioCBD+)
  - ○ BioCBD+'s Total Body Care Capsules
  - ○ Thrive (a pure CBD vape cartridge by VapeBright)
  - ○ Muscle and Joint Relief CBD Oil
- **ONNIT**
  - ○ New MOOD Daily Stress Formula
- **Four Sigmatic**
  - ○ All products are amazing, but my three favorites are Lions Mane (for brain boost), Reishi (for calming state), and Mushroom Coffee (for a big brain and body boost).

  Note: I'm an ambassador for some, but not all, of these companies. Go to http://www.ThisisTJ.com/FavoriteSupplements to access this list and consider trying some out for yourself.

We've tackled nutrition and supplements; now it's time to learn about mastering our movement.

Movement 101

Taking care of our bodies through proper physical movement is vitally important to overall health. But the problem is we must find the right balance of quantity and quality of movement. This is also our opportunity. No matter where you stand now, focusing on the *quality* of your movement is an important first step. I learned this the hard way.

When I moved to Miami to pursue modeling, I had just finished training as a High-Intensity Interval Training (H.I.I.T) group fitness instructor. Unfortunately, I didn't realize how hard it was on my body until following the workout program religiously for almost a year. And my body was paying the price. The workout program I was using was created to give a quick, powerful workout to people who want or need to stay at home to work out rather than going to the gym. It seems workout programs like this are popping up more and more all the time. Workouts that involve short bursts of high heart rate movement can work wonders for burning fat and staying fit, but we still need to focus on having a safe and effective movement session. For example, starting too fast, using improper form, or not incorporating enough rest into your routine can be hard on your body. Moreover, research data suggest that focusing exclusively on H.I.I.T. workouts may result in reduced enjoyment in that activity over time.

Thankfully, I've learned from my past experiences and evolved the way I approach movement and exercise altogether, seeking proper balance of the right type of functional movements.

So what's a healthy way to look at movement and exercise? As I shared earlier in the book, I was working out twice a day in Miami for the sole purpose of building a great-looking body for the cameras, not for optimal health and longevity. While it's OK to move your body and work out because you want to look good, don't forget the real reason for having a proper movement regimen: to gain and maintain strength, flexibility, and stability as we age. I have also tried to live out the idea of doing movement as a tribute to the body and the vital organs we possess. As the American professional boxer, Gene Tunney, once said, "Exercise should be regarded as a tribute to the heart."

I've blessed to learn from my mistakes with respect to movement and surround myself with a smart group of functional movement instructors who have given me feedback on my weaknesses, injuries, and overall approach to movement. With the right approach to movement, you too can develop habits that help you avoid pain and injury, as well as feel and look great—now and in the future.

Here are the main ways I've changed my approach to movement.

Ten Fundamental Ways I've Evolved My Movement Habits

1. Light movement and stretching in the morning
2. Move based on intuition and with ease
3. Let the breath guide the movement
4. Move more outside and less inside
5. Lift weights for function, not for vanity
6. Work on stability with Pilates
7. Make time for recreational movement with friends

8. Move in a fasted state
9. Engage in enjoyable physical activity and movement
10. Focus on posture and form

Light movement and stretching in the morning. When we wake up, our bodies are naturally a bit dehydrated from sleep. But, after we get a little water and sea salt, what do our bodies need most? Light movement to wake up the nervous system and get the blood flowing. As I start my day, I like to ease into physical activity to allow as much peace as possible to flow. That's why I usually do a light ten- to twenty-minute yoga or stretching routine, sometimes outside in the sun and sometimes in the comfort of my own home. This helps me get present in my body, feel what I'm feeling, and create a peaceful, balanced mind and body to start my day.

Move based on intuition and with ease. When I begin a movement session, I usually have a general plan of what I want to do and for how long; however, I also allow my intuition to flow. If I'm feeling like doing something different than I planned, I'll consider making a change or transition to something else. I'm also a fan of getting my heart rate up and working out hard, but I'm always mindful of doing so with ease.

Let the breath guide the movement. To support the first two movement objectives, I use my breath to guide my movement. Staying present with my breath and adding more intention to my inhales and exhales has brought a lot of peace to my movement routines.

Move more outside and less inside. Gyms and workout facilities all over the world have been created to make it more convenient for humans to workout. Unfortunately, this convenience has also contributed to our chronic disconnection with nature. Over the past few years, I've become a fan of moving my body outside as much as possible. Be it stretching, walking, cycling, or hiking—I'm able to get more fresh air, more connection with nature and sunlight outdoors, and less artificial blue light from being stuck indoors. Plus, I find that doing a movement session in nature allows me to check in with myself and stay balanced.

Lift weights for function, not for vanity. Strength training is a key area of movement to focus on, but doing it for the right reasons is also very important. I lift weights a few times a week. I love how it feels, I appreciate the strength it can build, and I believe the benefits of lifting weights will add years to my life. But I used to lift weights for the purpose of competing with others to see how much weight I could lift and to build muscles that looked good. This is not always a healthy mindset. Now I focus on lifting for function, not for vanity.

Work on stability with Pilates. When I first got into intentional movement, I didn't realize all the different areas of exercise to focus on, including strength, flexibility, and stability. Over time, my Pilates instructor, who also happens to be my girlfriend, has helped me add more stability-focused movement into my fitness routine. (Later, I'll share a fitness plan she helped me develop while writing this book.) I do mat work and work on a Pilates reformer machine. If you are interested in incorporating Pilates into your fitness routine, make sure you find a good instructor who knows what they're doing.

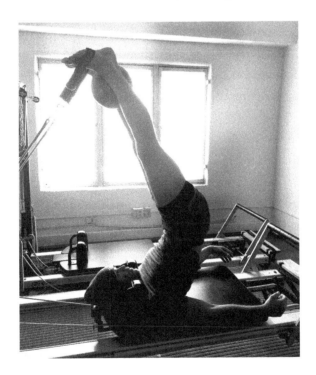

Make time for recreational movement with friends. Setting aside specific times during the week to move, sweat, and compete with friends can not only bring more accountability to your fitness, but also more fun. Some of my favorite recreational workouts include football, ultimate, and spikeball. If you haven't tried spikeball, it's worth checking out—super fun, engages your mind, and keeps you on your toes.

Move in a fasted state. One of the questions I often hear from people relates to eating and movement: "Should I move before or after I eat?" It depends on the person, the activity, and the goal of the activity. If you're looking to burn more fat while adding muscle, working out in a fasted state can help. I suggest people experiment with what works for them. This means not eating for at least two to four hours before your workout session (or at least approaching your workout session without too much food in your stomach). I enjoy how I feel lighter on my feet when moving in a fasted state, but again, experiment with what works for you.

Engage in enjoyable physical activity and movement. Enjoying your workouts is very important. If you are someone who could use more movement in your life, but you're having difficulty choosing or committing to an activity, consider starting with something you enjoy or have enjoyed in the past. This might be cycling, shooting hoops, or going for a walk—whatever is fun for you. That's what can keep you interested and motivated to keep moving your body. I would also add that just because you don't enjoy something now doesn't mean you can't enjoy it in the future. So try new things and you'll probably be surprised at how easy it can be to learn to enjoy a new practice.

Focus on posture and form. It may go without saying, but as you engage in your workouts, having good posture and form is incredibly important. If you want to experience the best results while also avoiding injury, learning the correct form and getting feedback is a smart approach. If you have any friends or colleagues in the fitness space, consider getting their feedback on your form. Or, you can also research proper posture and form on your own. Just make sure to seek a nice balance of self-learning and expert-led training.

These are the core principles I've used to evolve my integrative approach to movement. If you're interested in seeing a more in-depth fitness plan, check out the following breakdown of muscles to strengthen and muscles to lengthen, as suggested by Amanda Gyuran, my girlfriend and Pilates trainer. *Note:* The following fitness plan is specific to me and gets super scientific. I don't expect you to understand everything in this plan, nor should you follow this plan on your own.

Example of TJ's Fitness Plan

Muscles to Strengthen:

- Adductors (inner thighs) to help prevent knee pain
- Abductors (specifically glute medius and minimus) to prevent knee/hip pain and aid in pelvic stabilization
- Multifidus for overall core strength and spinal stabilization as well as prevention for any lumbar spine or hip pain
- Obliques (both external and internal) to aid in better spinal mobility
- Serratus Anterior (the pushing muscle) to prevent "winging," aid in scapular stability, and help with elbow, forearm, and hand pain, as well as cervical spine injuries
- Rhomboids, Low Traps, Latissimus Dorsi, Teres minor, and Teres major to aid in scapular stability
- Triceps Brachii (strengthen all three—long head, medial head, and lateral head—but especially the long head and lateral head) to protect the radial and ulnar nerve and help with elbow, forearm, and hand pain
- Lower Cervical Extensors (splenius cervicis, semispinalis cervicis, and longissimus cervicis) to correct forward head and address cervical spine injuries
- Upper Cervical (Capital) Flexors (longus capitis, rectus capitis anterior, and suprahyoid muscles) to correct forward head and address cervical spine injuries

Muscles to Lengthen (stretch while maintaining strength):

- Piriformis to prevent hip pain/popping
- Lower Cervical Flexors (sternocleidomastoid, anterior, and medial scalene muscles) to correct forward head and address cervical spine injuries

- Upper Cervical (Capital) Extensors (semispinalis capitis, longissimus capitis, splenius capitis, and suboccipital muscles) to correct forward head and address cervical spine injuries
- Psoas, Sartorius, and Hamstrings

Moving on, we have one last core area of our health to focus on—our sleep.

Sleep 101

What is the goal of sleep? For me, it is to get enough quantity of sleep and have proper quality sleep that when I wake up, I feel refreshed, clear minded, and energized for the day.

Sleep is our time to rest, regenerate, and recover from the day. But to get great sleep, we don't just need to focus on going to bed on time or our evening and morning routines. It's also important to look at how our behaviors and access to sunlight affect our ability to get great sleep.

The amount of sunlight you receive during the day has a big impact on your circadian system—the internal clock that helps control numerous processes in the body. Sunlight exposure signals your hypothalamus (an area of the brain that is the master gland of your hormonal system) and all corresponding organs and glands to wake up. It triggers your body to produce proper levels of the hormones and chemical messengers that regulate your internal clock. These include both serotonin (crucial in regulating your body's clock) and cortisol (the hormone that gives us the energy to wake up).

Like proper sunlight, there are several other areas of our lifestyle that impact our ability to get quality sleep. And, thankfully, over the past few years, I've discovered some key strategies to improve the quality of my sleep.

In this section, I'll share the top ten ways I've evolved my sleep habits and we'll explore some key areas of our day that impact our sleep.

Ten Fundamental Ways I've Evolved My Sleep Habits

1. Darken the room with blackout shades
2. Create a sleep sanctuary
3. Use blue blocker sunglasses

4. Set an optimal temperature
5. Get a quality mattress and pillow
6. Avoid certain foods and drinks before bed
7. Set a bedtime and work backward
8. Create a sacred evening routine
9. Use specific supplements
10. Hack your snooze and study your sleep

Darken the room with blackout shades. Getting great sleep has a lot to do with optimizing our circadian rhythms. And one of the easiest ways to do that is to create an environment that is pitch-black at night. Can you see light coming from outside while you sleep? Even a little bit of light can disrupt your ability to get quality, deep sleep. That's why I suggest you find some sort of black out curtains or shades to use while you're sleeping at night. I found a great set from Bed Bath & Beyond, but you can probably do a Google or Amazon search to find some other great options. Trust me, once you use black-out curtains, you'll never want to go back.

Create a sleep sanctuary. In addition to making your room feel like a dark cave, it can also be helpful to create a sleep sanctuary environment in your room. For example, you could get a pink Himalayan salt lamp, an essential oil diffuser, or calming wall art to hang around your room. It's also important to keep technology out of the bedroom—during the day, but most importantly, at night.

Use blue blocker sunglasses. For the past two years, I've been using blue-light-blocking sunglasses. Why? To get better sleep and live longer. Many intentional health hackers realize the importance of light regulation for the human body, but the question is, how do we hack it? While there are several important parts of different colors of light (and different spectrums of each color), one important and simple hack is to block as much artificial blue light during the afternoon and evening as possible. Thomas Edison and Nikola Tesla made some major moves back in the day with the invention of the light bulb. But, unfortunately, we're paying a price: fewer candles and fires mean more bright, artificial blue light from our light bulbs and screens. What's wrong with blue light, you may wonder? According to several studies, blue light disrupts melatonin production, which affects the brain and body's ability to get enough quality sleep. Plus, it tells the brain and body it's not nighttime. I own a few pairs of blue-blocker sunglasses, but my favorite ones are "Swannies" from Swanwick Sleep, because they're pretty stylish. My friend James Swanwick created these to help people block blue light at night and look good doing it.

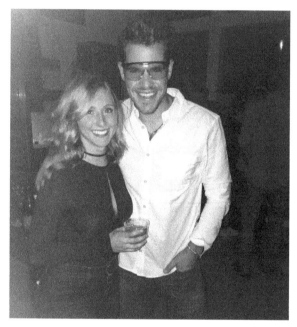

Wearing blue blocker sunglasses at a Paleo Fx Conference after-party in Austin, Texas, with my girlfriend, Amanda.

Set an optimal temperature. Depending on the weather outside, I prefer to keep the temperature in the house and my bedroom at around 69°F while I'm sleeping. But more than that, I prefer to go to bed not feeling warm or hot. It's impossible for me to get to sleep and stay asleep if I'm too warm. That's why I'll sometimes take a warm to cold shower before bed. That's also why I usually sleep naked. So if you're struggling with quality of sleep, make sure you consider your ideal body and room temperature.

Get a quality mattress and pillow. This may go without saying, but the quality of your mattress and pillow really makes a difference in the quality of your sleep. The key to mattress shopping is to find one that feels comfortable, but you also want to look out for the environment and your health. Many mattresses are known to have chemicals pouring out of them, which is the last thing you want to breathe in all night while you sleep. I suggest finding organic mattress and pillow companies that take comfort into account, of course, but also healthy, clean, chemical-free materials. (*Note*: I'm a big fan of SAMINA, an organic mattress company based out of Austria. With their US headquarters based in Pasadena, California, I met the SAMINA team at one of the health conferences I attended a few years ago and nearly fell asleep on their bed in a room filled with hundreds of people.) The bottom line: Don't settle for a cheap mattress or pillow. I made this mistake once, and I won't make it again. I plan to order a SAMINA very soon. After all, we spend about a third of our lives in bed, so we may as well invest in a high-quality mattress and pillow.

Avoid certain foods and drinks before bed. When we prepare for bed, it's very important to take hunger levels and what we eat into account. After all, our brains require a little bit of glucose to achieve high-quality sleep. But the key is choosing foods and drinks that will help, not harm, your overall sleep quality. Some examples of drinks you may want to avoid for at least three to four hours before bed include, but are not limited to, any sort of alcoholic, caffeinated, or sugary beverage. Some examples of foods to avoid, include, but are not limited to, high-glycemic carbohydrates (e.g., breads, pizza, pasta) and anything with too much salt. No one likes waking up puffy from food choices made the night before. I like to go to bed on a semi-full stomach. Basically, I like to eat dinner about three to four hours before bed, and sometimes I'll have a late-night snack, such as cherries, almonds, or maybe a dash of local raw honey. Cherries have high melatonin content, a crucial hormone that helps regulate sleep and wake cycles. Almonds are high in calcium, which supports melatonin production, and are semi-filling, thanks to their fat and protein content. And honey? Honey doesn't just taste great; if you use local, raw honey and only have 1–2 teaspoons before bed, it can be a great way to give your brain enough glucose to use as energy while you sleep.

Set a bedtime and work backward. One of the keys to getting good sleep is making sure you don't just get quality sleep, but also enough sleep. So if you want to get an optimal quantity of sleep, ask yourself what time you want to wake up the next morning and work backward to set your bedtime accordingly. For example, let's say you want to get eight hours of sleep every night. And you want (or need) to be awake by 6:30 a.m. the next morning. That means you would need to sleep from 10:30 p.m. to 6:30 a.m. to achieve your goal of eight hours. Remember, it's important to make sure you start your bedtime routine BEFORE the time you need to be asleep. I like to be in bed about fifteen to twenty minutes before I want to fall asleep to give myself some time to fall asleep naturally. The last thing you want is to be rushed before you go to sleep. So keep it simple, and choose your wake and bed time wisely.

Create a sacred evening routine. In your quest to setting a bedtime and getting high quality sleep, it's important to look at the routine you follow before bed. When I approach my evening routine with the intention of peace and relaxation, it allows my mind and body to start to relax and get ready for bed naturally. Yes, we may have our standard habits of brushing our teeth and washing our face, but we can also find other ways to create a sacred evening routine. Consider doing a light stretch and peaceful breathing while listening to some relaxing music. And if your mind is still racing for some reason, you can consider doing a quick journal or meditation session before bed. If you want the highest quality of sleep possible, it's up to you to choose the relaxing habits and routines you want to get ready for bed.

Use specific supplements. Throughout this book, I've talked about the role of specific supplements to aid in stress management as well as energy and focus during your day. But these same supplements can work wonders to help you relax and be blessed with a high quality of sleep. Consider trying one or more of the supplements or drinks mentioned in chapter 10 (e.g., CBD, chamomile tea, lavender tea, Reishi mushrooms, Kava) an hour or so before bed. You'll be glad you did.

Hack your snooze and study your sleep. Last, but not least on my top-ten list for improving my sleep, is focusing on our relationship with the almighty snooze button. I'll be the first to admit hitting the snooze button happens a lot in my life. And that's OK. The key isn't to avoid hitting the snooze button altogether, but to listen to your body when your alarm does go off and see if it's ready to wake. If you have some time to spare, it may serve you to sleep a bit longer. But you'll want to make sure you avoid the costly mistake of going back to bed.

One of the ultimate sleep hacks is to measure the quality of your sleep. I'm not usually a big fan of wearables due to their potentially harmful Electromagnetic Frequency (EMF) Waves (from Bluetooth) looking to send information to your device. But for those who want to experiment with using a wearable to study their sleep, I would recommend trying out the Oura Ring. I haven't personally used one yet, but I've talked to several people who have, as well as a member of the Oura Ring team, to learn about how they work. The Oura Ring is worn on one of your fingers, which may allow for more accurate readings than if worn on your wrist. The Oura Ring is also one of the only wearables constantly tracking your HRV data (covered in chapter 11), and has an "airplane mode" that allows you to turn off Bluetooth while you sleep, while still collecting data. It's currently the only wearable I'm suggesting people try, and I plan to order one soon.

So there you have it—thirty tips in the areas of sleep, movement, and nutrition based on my own personal experience.

Your Daily Routine

In closing this chapter, as you look to experiment with ways of optimizing these areas of your health, I would first suggest you run through the following exercise to take an inventory of your current daily routine. Identify your priorities and put these priorities into action within your daily routine.

With the responsibilities of family and work potentially competing with our health goals, it becomes very important to create a system that allows us to stay focused and clear minded. Enter the 80/20 system, also known as the Pareto principle, where focusing on 20 percent of inputs is responsible for 80 percent of results. When I asked Ben Greenfield how he applies the 80/20 principle to his health goals and daily routine, this is how he responded:

> Set up a system where when you wake up in the morning, you know the daily theme in terms of what you will achieve professionally and personally. That's worked really well for me. It helps me to keep a clear

head and wake up in the morning with confidence about what I'll do that day.

This approach is a great way to compartmentalize your day—professionally and personally—but also to integrate your daily goals, so your professional and personal goals receive equal focus throughout your day. Often we neglect our health because we're too focused on our work or business. If that applies to you, then the simple approach Greenfield suggests could be a great strategy for you to try.

To close this chapter, I'll leave you with one more recommendation—not from me, but from health and nutrition expert JJ Virgin—about the top health hacks she would recommend for people to become more well-rounded, health-conscious consumers. Her answer was simple, yet powerful:

> The best health hack of all things possible is a journal. Don't overwhelm yourself. Pick one thing. Pick the first health hack you will do. Whether it's related to water, sleep, or vitamins, just start somewhere and journal every day with your big intention in mind.

The simplicity of her answer is what I love the most—pick one thing and journal every day. Sometimes self-care can be as simple as a little reflective journal exercise. You never know what kind of clarity you can create until you journal about your state.

Summary:
- You don't have to be a nutritionist or dietitian to learn about nutrition. You just need to find a strong enough interest and motivation to learn and experiment.
- The **Cycling Principle** suggests you cycle on and off specific nutrition or supplement habits over time. Cycling on and off specific types of vitamins, minerals, and other ingredients allows our brain, body, and entire biochemical process to take a break from certain variables so as not to become dependent or too used to them.

- Nootropics are supplements specifically designed to help enhance cognitive function in some way—boosting our real-time ability to focus, manage our memory, or activate a more creative state.
- It's OK to move your body and work out because you want to look good. But don't forget the real reason for having a proper movement regimen—to gain and maintain strength, flexibility, and stability as we age.
- What is the goal of sleep? Personally, I want to get enough quantity of sleep and have proper quality sleep so when I wake up, I feel refreshed, clear minded, and energized for the day.
- With the responsibilities of family and work potentially competing with your health goals, it becomes very important to create a system that allows you to give equal focus to all parts of your life. Consider setting personal health goals and professional goals for each part of your day.

Action Items:

1. Journal and reflect on your current approach to nutrition.
    - Are there certain changes you think would be helpful for your nutrition strategy?
    - How can you evolve your relationship with nutrition and supplements?
    - Are there any supplements you are curious about trying?
    - Take a look at the ten ways I've evolved my nutrition habits and choose a few new habits to try out yourself. (Remember to consult your health care team before trying a new diet or supplements.)

2. Journal and reflect on your current approach to movement.
    - How can you evolve your relationship with movement?
    - Can you move more? If so, what movements would you choose?
    - Do you need to move less? Do you have any injuries that need to heal or be looked at by a medical professional?
    - Can you get outside and reconnect with nature?
    - Can you focus more on movement that you love and enjoy?

- Take a look at the ten ways I've evolved my movement habits and choose a few new habits to try out yourself.

3. Reflect on your current approach to sleep.
   - How can you evolve your relationship with sleep?
   - Are you getting enough sleep?
   - What does your evening routine look like?
   - Take a look at the top ten ways I've evolved my sleep habits, and choose a few new habits to try out yourself.

4. Let's apply Ben Greenfield's strategy of knowing what you want to achieve personally and professionally each day by asking yourself the following questions:
   - What are a few personal health goals to focus on in the morning, afternoon, and evening?
   - What are a few professional goals to focus on in the morning, afternoon, and evening?
   - Your mental or written list may look something like this:

   Morning
   Personal Health Goals:
   Professional Goals:

   Afternoon
   Personal Health Goals:
   Professional Goals:

   Evening Goals
   Personal Health Goals:
   Professional Goals:

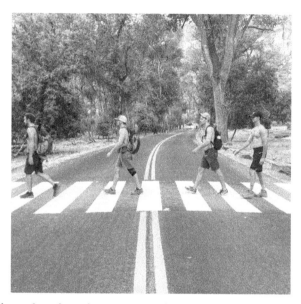

With my friends, Joshua, Peter, and Stefan, on our way to hike in Zion National Park near Springdale, Utah. Photo credit: Todd Murphy

CHAPTER 15

Nature, Music, and Enjoying the Ride

One touch of nature makes the whole world kin.
– William Shakespeare

There is a reason people report being happier and healthier in certain cities and states across America. Your environment matters. And, perhaps most importantly, your relationship with your environment matters.

There are a lot of areas for us to focus on when taking a holistic health hacker approach. We've covered a lot of these areas throughout this book, including our relationships with family, friends, as well as our spiritual relationships with God and the divine. But what about God's other powerful creation—planet Earth?

This book is about inspiring people to become a bit more artful in their approach to their health and their lives in general. And art involves creative action. So as we close this book, I'd like to discuss nature and music, two of the more creative parts of our environment that can play a surprisingly important role in our overall health and happiness.

Consider the following questions:

- Could we leverage both nature and music to support us in our health and performance goals? If so, how?
- What is it about nature and music that can move mountains, so to speak, inside the hearts and souls of humans?
- Can we create the state we desire on command just by pressing play on certain types of music?

Both nature and music are inexpensive, easy ways of changing our environment to activate a desired state. It's time we explore these areas a bit more to see how they can complement our lives in the best possible way.

Nature for the Win

I have been blessed to travel to beautiful places in our country, like Florida and Colorado—visiting the beach and mountains seems extra special when you grow up around corn and soybean fields. I was even lucky enough to travel out of the country a few times: a choir trip to Italy in high school, a visit to Germany and France during college, and a ski trip to Japan after college. But my deep love for nature wasn't fully realized until my visit to Zion National Park in Utah during the summer of 2016.

Several San Diego based friends and I had just completed a four-day entrepreneurship conference at a hotel in Las Vegas. We were tired of the sound of slot machines and the artificial blue light confusing our circadian rhythms. Instead, we were craving time in the sunshine amid the great outdoors.

There were five of us in my friend Peter's Jeep, headed east for a four-day adventure. Only one of us had been to Zion before, but all of us knew it was going to be special. As some high-performance experts would say, we had what's referred to as "group flow" on our sides. Meaning, we had shared goals and were all equally leading this epic adventure together. We were in a synchronistic flow state of sorts—feeling and performing at our best in an effortless way. So much so, that we consciously made a group decision to take a break from our smartphones. We decided to disconnect from technology and social media, agreeing to put our phones in airplane mode and live 100 percent in the present moment.

We called it our "Get Off the Grid" trip—the "grid" being the internet. In a world where more and more people are tethered to their smartphones, taking an intentional break from these devices, social media, and the internet in general can bring a lot of peace, relaxation, and adventure.

Now, were all five of us 100 percent compliant with our no phone/no internet policy throughout this trip? Nope. We relied on our phones for GPS while driving to new places and our camera when we wanted to capture a moment for posterity. But we did take a complete break from social media, as well as email and texting, and reaped the benefits of time well spent in nature.

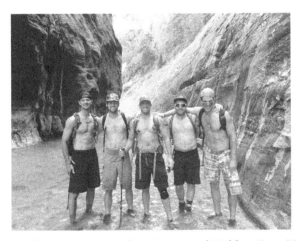

"Off the Grid" with Stefan, Joshua, Peter, and Todd in Zion National Park.

During this trip, we wondered if any other hikers had considered the importance of taking a break from technology as we had. At the top of Angels Landing, one of the more popular (and dangerous) trails in Zion, there is the most epic view. But in looking down, we couldn't help but notice other hikers on their phones during most of their hike. At times, we saw more people on their smartphones than not. We called these people "Gridders" because it seemed like they couldn't disconnect from the grid of social media or the internet. (But, hey, at least they were outside on technology, not glued to their devices inside an office building.) Likewise, whenever one of us would use our smartphone for some reason (even if it was just for a quick photo), we would all get called out as a "Gridder" as well.

All joking aside, the topic of technology versus nature is real and important if we want to evolve our culture in the healthiest way possible.

As previously discussed in chapter 10, APA's (2017) Stress in America survey data suggest that while many Americans (65 percent) report taking a break from technology is important to their mental health, very few of those individuals (28 percent) actually do.

So why is there a nearly 40 percent gap between people who want to take a break and those who actually do? Why don't we do what improves our mental health and makes us happy, like spending more time in nature away from the digital world?

Researchers, may have found an answer. In experiments testing anticipated and actual experiences, Nisbet and Zelenski found that, on average, people tend to underestimate how good they will feel after having brief contact with nature. Social scientists call these bad predictions *forecasting errors*. As it turns out, people may choose not to spend much time in nature because their chronic disconnection from nature causes them to underestimate nature's health benefits.

It seems that we, as humans, are quickly losing our historically strong connection with nature. As of 2008, for the first time ever, the world's population was evenly split between urban and rural areas. Urbanization, which refers to the shift from rural to urban areas, has continued its momentum. As of 2017, more people live in an urban setting than a rural setting. In addition to this trend of living further and further from nature, and sometimes independent of where we live, there are consequences from the lack of time we are spending outdoors getting fresh air and sunlight.

For example, according to data from the US Centers for Disease Control and Prevention (CDC) National Health and Nutrition Examination Survey, nearly one in ten children has a Vitamin D deficiency. That's 7.6 million children. And another 50.8 million are considered Vitamin D insufficient, perhaps due to limited time spent outdoors.

As I shared earlier, seeking Vitamin D from the sun is one reason I bought a one-way flight to California in the middle of an Iowa winter. But more than my levels of a particular vitamin, my mind, body, and all of my senses felt like they were missing something after my experience in Zion. Our "Get Off The Grid" adventure really did inspire a new love affair with nature. After noticing changes in my energy and overall levels of stress after this trip, I realized how intentional time in nature could help me live a healthier and happier life. So much so, that since writing this book, I moved to California for six months to live near the beach and later to Boulder, Colorado, in order to live near the mountains. Something about the beach and the mountains were calling my name. It just *felt* right. I don't have a lot of quantifiable data beyond that feeling. Instead, I simply responded to my intuition of what I was called to do, and consciously decided where I wanted to live based on how I wanted to feel and spend my time. I was craving nature time! It's just that simple.

If nature can provide this much benefit to me, and even inspire me to move to a whole new city and state, then it is not at all surprising that researchers are focused on studying the benefits of nature.

In *The Nature Fix: Why Nature Makes us Happier, Healthier, and More Creative,* author Florence Williams explores the benefits of nature with the help of top researchers who measure the quantitative health benefits of nature. Williams recounts her personal journey of leaving the mountains for city life when she moved from Boulder, Colorado, to Washington, D.C. It was after this move that she realized how we, as a society, take nature for granted:

> Yet we think of nature as a luxury, not a necessity. We don't recognize how much it elevates us, both personally and politically. That, ultimately, is the aspiration of this book: to find the best science behind our nature-primed neurons and to share it.

As a journalist who frequently writes about nature, Williams starts her quest-of-a-book off with a story of her own travel experiences in Japan, taking part in what the Japanese call "forest bathing." Forest bathing, or *Shinrin-yoku* in Japanese, is a real thing people do specifically for the benefits of time spent in nature—not physically bathing in any sort of liquid, but simply spending leisure time in the forest. As Williams goes on to explain in her book,

The Japanese go crazy for this practice, which is standard preventive medicine here. It involves cultivating your senses to open them to the woods. It's not about wilderness; it's about the nature/civilization hybrid the Japanese have cultivated for thousands of years.

This is an important point for us all to consider. We don't necessarily need to become mountain men or wilderness women to receive all the health benefits of nature. We just need to find a middle-ground approach that involves intentional time spent in nature. We can learn from countries like Japan that go to great lengths to provide data about the benefits of nature to the world.

Japan, whose forests cover 68 percent of the country's landmass, has funded nearly $4 million in forest-bathing research through Japan's Forest Agency since 2003. They have forty-eight official Forest Therapy trails designated for this practice. To support these efforts, Japan also has a handful of physicians certified in forest medicine and local cabins placed near their forest therapy trails to measure changes in important biomarkers (e.g., blood pressure, heart rate, and cortisol levels) before and after a visit to the forest. And the data checks out. As Williams shares in her book, researchers conducting field studies in Japanese forest sites have found that viewing and walking in forest areas resulted in better moods and lower anxiety, and produced greater changes in several physiological states when compared with viewing and walking in urban areas. In fact, simply viewing forest areas resulted in a 12 percent decrease in cortisol levels, a 7 percent decrease in sympathetic nerve activity, a 1.4 percent decrease in blood pressure, and a nearly 6 percent decrease in heart rate.

I highly recommend checking out Williams' book if you are interested in reading more about this topic or want to dive deeper into her story.

In order to understand the importance and benefits of time spent in nature, we also need to understand the potential downsides of not spending enough time in nature. Some refer to this phenomenon as "Nature-Deficit Disorder," a term coined by journalist Richard Louv in his 2005 book, *Last Child in the Woods*. Louv uses the term to give meaning to our changing relationship with nature; specifically, how we as human beings, especially children, are spending less quality time outdoors, resulting in a wide range of mental and behavior problems.

I can't imagine a more important topic than our relationship with nature. This is how I see it—technology is a tool. Nature is our habitat. So if we're interested in creating a healthy relationship with technology, we must master our relationship with our environment first. If we don't take advantage of the benefits time spent in nature can bring *without* technology, we're missing out on an essential aspect of life.

In April 2017, I hosted an experiential health hacking event called Elevate Your State LIVE. Putting technology aside to experience nature was a big part of my message at this event, so much so that we did a parkour workout outside at a local park and ended the second day with a sunset hike and farm-to-table meal at the top of a mountain.

Put simply, the idea that we all need to get outside more is an important message worth spreading. From a short walk to the park to a hike in a major national forest, there are a lot of ways to spend time in nature. If you're ready to spend some more time in nature, but not sure where to start or how to go about it, **consider the following tips to elevate your experience in nature:**

1. Set your intention.

Before getting out in nature, do a little preparation to see where you want to go and how much time you have to spend. It's important to set your intention so you know WHY you're spending time in nature and HOW you want to feel during and after your time spent in nature.

2. Do it by yourself.

Consider spending time in nature by yourself first, maybe for a twenty- to thirty-minute walk. If done right, nature provides peace and quiet that allows your mind to unwind and your body to breathe deeply.

3. Do it with friends.

After you explore nature by yourself, try spending time in nature with friends or family. Interacting with those closest to you in this way can support your efforts of deepening relationships. Plus, like I experienced with my friends in Zion, it can bring some added fun and group flow.

4. Pack Wisely.

Bring high quality food and water, stay hydrated with spring water and sea salt, and consider bringing a book or journal. You never know when the moment will spark a creative idea or point of self-reflection.

5. Gear Up.

Depending on the level of your nature adventure, make sure you have the proper gear. I would suggest you at least have a strong pair of hiking shoes, but it's worth looking into other gear, such as a proper bag and clothing. Check out your local outdoor clothing and equipment store, or a national brand such as Patagonia or REI.

6. Don't plan everything.

Having a general plan for your time spent in nature can be helpful and important, but so can going with the flow. Allowing for some flow and creativity in your nature quest allows you to practice being unattached to the moment. This way you'll find and notice things that were unexpected and would have gone unappreciated.

7. Reflect on how you feel.

After you finish your nature adventure, make sure you reflect on your overall experience. Explore how you feel and what you experienced. Nature can speak to you if you're open to engaging your senses to listen. You could also consider measuring changes in resting heart rate, HRV, or blood pressure, if you'd like.

Now that we've covered the role of nature in our lives, let's transition to another key area of artful health hacking—our relationship with music.

Music that Moves You

Music is one of my favorite art forms. In fact, it was one of the first art forms I ever really enjoyed. I sang in middle school choir (because we had to) and in high school choir (because I wanted to). Since then, I've become a connoisseur of music, more for the benefits I receive as a listener than as a singer on stage.

From helping us process emotions to bringing us closer together, there are a lot of different ways music impacts our lives. Can it help us relax? Can it give us energy? Can it motivate us to take action or help us change certain behaviors? The answer, based on my personal experiences, is a big fat yes.

And what role does music play in our health? Let's take a peek at the science of sound and, specifically, the ways in which music can affect our brains, bodies, and even our relationships with friends and family.

In the book *This is Your Brain on Music: The Science of a Human Obsession*, Dr. Daniel Levitin explores the connection between music—how it works and why we listen to it—and the human brain. Levitin also partnered with Sonos (the smart speaker manufacturer) and Apple to explore the role of music in our homes and lives.

In this joint research study, thirty thousand music listeners from eight different countries were surveyed about the role music plays in their lives. Thirty homes and 109 participants from the eight countries were selected to participate in a two-week field study. For the first week, members of those thirty households were instructed to avoid listening to music out loud. The following week, however, participants could listen to as much music out loud as they wanted. In fact, the researchers supported their music-listening efforts by providing each home with a Sonos sound system to play Apple Music, Apple Watches, iPhones (to function with the Apple Watch, collect data, and allow for video journaling), Nest Cams, and iBeacons (a broadcaster beacon device to send data and information to a receiver or smartphone app). Quite the gifts of advanced technology in the name of research!

By observing people in the natural habitat of their own homes, researchers were able to gain a unique perspective of the impact music has in the daily lives of individuals and families. One of the notable findings involved the proximity of the music listeners. When music was playing at home, people moved physically closer together. (The average distance between household members decreased by 12 percent during the study.) In an interview with John Paul Titlow from the magazine *Fast Company*, Levitin referred to this as "a nexus of intimacy and togetherness."

Additionally, with music playing, people were 33 percent more likely to cook together and 85 percent more likely to invite people over. Among the initial thirty thousand music listeners surveyed by Sonos, couples reported 66 percent more intimacy when music is playing. And in the home experiment, a related phenomenon was observed—couples spent 37 percent more "awake time" in bed, and I don't believe they were working on their taxes.

As Levitin explains, there's a neurochemical basis for these findings. Listening to music out loud triggers the release of the hormones oxytocin (the love hormone) and serotonin (impacts our mood, sleep, and sex-drive). You could say that music, when played out loud, enhances the overall human experience. Put simply, there is a different kind of music to help motivate, inspire, or enhance the joy you experience during different activities. In his interview with Titlow, Levitin explains,

> We find from studies that people listen to a different kind of music when they're cleaning the house. Then there's a different kind of music to help motivate you through your exercise workout. The same way we use coffee to get stimulated or alcohol or pot to get calm, we have music that fits these different moods or alters these different moods and alters their neurochemistry.

Plus, with music playing in the background, more dance parties will break which means more physical activity and fluid movement. I'd be lying if I said I haven't busted out some dance moves while jamming to some tunes at the gym. Music makes life and workouts more fun!

Lastly, according to the Sonos study, respondents who listened to music were about 25 percent less irritable and 25 percent more inspired. They reported a 16 percent increase in positive feelings overall. These findings demonstrate that music can not only bring us closer to our loved ones, but also add an overall sense of positivity, inspiration, and joy to our lives.

So, how can we, as health hackers, experiment with new ways of using music in our lives, adding a bit more intention to the type and timing of music we play? How can we optimize our relationship with music in order to bring about more love, health, and joy in our lives? What are some ways we can experiment with using the right music to support our health and performance?

Music is not something we have to passively listen to; rather, we can create and curate music on our own. With online services like Spotify, Soundcloud, YouTube, and iTunes, there is no shortage of platforms with which to design our musical experience.

Don't be afraid to let the music lead you. I have several go-to songs and playlists based on my state. For example, if I am getting tired and it is close to bedtime, I can play some calm music, such as Jack Johnson, *Chillout Radio* on Spotify, or the *Garden State* soundtrack. While my taste in music may be different than yours, I'm betting you are able to find a calming musician, group, song, or playlist on your favorite music platform (e.g., Soundcloud, Spotify, YouTube).

Lyrics or No Lyrics?

In the past few years, I've found music without lyrics or words can bring a lot more effortless flow, peace, and productivity to my lifestyle. This non-lyrical music (played out loud or through headphones) can create greater depth to our experience. At least it has for me.

Here are some examples of the non-lyrical music tools I use to support my healing, level of stress, and ability to stay grounded and focused in my work on a daily basis:

- Brain.fm
- Wholetones
- Calm.com
- YouTube, Spotify, and Soundcloud

Brain.fm. Brian.fm uses an online membership platform to provide different types of non-lyrical music designed to help you create different brain states, such as focus, relaxation, or sleep. Brain.fm has designed a very simple system combining music with auditory neuroscience to produce an innovative non-invasive digital therapy application for consumers. Leveraging artificial intelligence, Brain.fm composes unique music just for you and the state you want to create. In my experience, this stuff flat out works.

Wholetones. Another favorite source of music for me is a musical soundtrack called *Wholetones: The Healing Frequency Music Project*. It is a collection of seven, twenty-two minute audio sessions (songs), each resonating at a unique frequency aimed at addressing a specific area of healing in our bodies. In my experience, all seven non-lyrical songs provide a beautiful sound to my ears and a deep sense of relaxation and peace, as well as emotional and spiritual healing. Don't believe me? Check out their Amazon reviews and ratings. Begin by taking their free quiz about your health and causes of stress. Based on my answers, I resonate with a 639 HZ frequency, which corresponds to their song *The Bridge*. According to their website, this song fosters forgiveness and peace in relationships, which can contribute to a stronger immune system and less stress on adrenal glands.

Calm.com. The first app I ever used for mindfulness and relaxation was Calm. The Calm app provides a tool to calm the mind and add more mindfulness into your day. I haven't used the app for a while, but it's definitely worth looking into. I believe they have a free trial and paid versions of the app.

YouTube, Spotify, and Soundcloud. I grouped these three options together as they are very similar, large-scale music, audio, and video platforms. I'll often play some long, non-lyrical ambient music by Tycho, or even cue up some hour-long Wholetones audio recordings that have been posted on YouTube. My favorite YouTube song is called "Youthing." On Spotify and Soundcloud, I like to create playlists based on the time of day or the state I want to create. I also like Spotify channels specifically designed to support certain states (e.g., focus, relaxation). Whether you already use one or more of these platforms or haven't tried one yet, we can all add a bit more intention and focus to the types of music we use music to support our health.

As a side note, music can be a great support tool, but it's also not necessarily something to become dependent on. For example, I have noticed in the past that music was becoming a crutch during a movement session. I found it harder to move if I didn't have my music, as if music was my trigger in a healthy habit loop. For the past several months, I've been experimenting with moving *without* music and I really love it. Additionally, listening to energizing music can put me in an over-energized state at times, to the point that I lose peace and presence in the body.

Silence, even from the sound of nature, can sometimes surprise your senses and give you exactly what you need—the ability to listen to your body. I suggest you find your happy medium with respect to music and observe the benefits in your own life.

Protect Yourself

Now that we've covered the role of music and our environment in enhancing our health, I'd like to explore a few ways you can protect yourself from potentially harmful elements of these topics. As mentioned in chapter 14, there are certain technologies, such as wearable watches, rings, and other devices, that can help us hack and track our health and add value to our lives. Additionally, we've talked a lot about the importance of having an intentional relationship with our smartphones and other devices. But to close the book, I want to leave you with a few more small action steps that may help protect you and your family.

Note: I'm not a scientific expert on this topic. This is simply an area of my health that I've been learning more about the past few years. I suggest you do your own research and, ultimately, make a decision about how you want to approach this topic.

1. Invest in a radiation-blocking cell phone and laptop case.

At the beginning of this book, I briefly referenced how I was blocking the radiation from my cell phone with a phone case made by a company named SafeSleeve. I first learned about SafeSleeve in an article written by Ben Greenfield, and have been using their products ever since.

In response to concerns about electromagnetic radiation (EMR) exposure, SafeSleeve created cell phone, tablet, and laptop cases that shield the user from three types of EMR—extremely low frequencies, radio frequencies (e.g., Wi-Fi), and thermal radiation (heat). According to SafeSleeve's website, a growing number of doctors and scientists are warning that prolonged exposure to EMR increases our risk of various diseases, and the EPA has labeled EMFs a "class 3 carcinogen."

I used to fear putting my laptop on my lap while working or having my phone in my pocket right next to my nether region. Not anymore. I love that their phone cases have a tiny hole for audio output and input, allowing you to easily take phone calls and listen to music while the case is closed. If you like using your phone, but don't like the idea of exposure to potentially harmful radiation, check out SafeSleeve's website: https://www.safesleevecases.com/.

2. Turn off your wireless internet at night.

Every night before I go to bed, I unplug my router from the wall outlet. While there are mixed views on the health impact of radio frequency technology, who really needs the internet while they sleep? Having your router on at night provides no value to your sleep routine, and several people I personally know suggest that it impacts their sleep and overall health. This is a simple step to add to your bedtime routine, and depending on your current state, may help you sleep better.

3. Pick up a pair of Dr. Mercola's Blue Tube headphones.

As previously discussed in this chapter, music can provide major benefits to our health and relationships. And if you're like me, you may sometimes listen to music using headphones. But if we're using headphones, we want to make sure we're using the right ones—headphones that will protect us while still delivering a high quality audio experience.

While writing this book, I ran an experiment on myself to see how I responded to two different types of headphones. The first pair was over the ear headphones that I had heard could help restore long term hearing function, and the second pair was a Blue Tube Headset that uses in-ear tubes designed to block out nearly all of the radio frequencies associated with whatever device you may be using. And the results for me, in my N=1 experiment, were clear—I felt much better with the Blue Tube headset. Something about having large headphones over my ears created a feeling of heat and energy around my ears and cheekbones that seemed to add to my stress. The Blue Tube headphones were much different. They were light and didn't put too much weight or pressure on my ears or my body. Plus, the sound quality was great. I now use these headphones for pretty much everything—from listening to music while working or working out, to taking phone calls. Learn more at http://products.mercola.com/blue-tube-headset/.

Find Joy in Your Journey

Throughout this book, we've touched on many areas of our health with a focus on leveraging the latest principles of sustainable behavior change to make improvements. If we want to grow in our health, energy, and overall lifestyle, we must make some kind of change. But sustainable behavior change rarely happens without one thing—**finding the joy.** In order to blossom, grow, or improve, we must cultivate some level of joy.

To close, I invite you to consider how you can find more joy in your health journey:

- What brings you joy in your life? For example, what do you already enjoy in terms of food, fitness, and time spent in nature?
- Does the joy you experience in these activities keep you focused and encouraged?
- How can you build more joy into your life and your health?
- Let your heart lead you and your joy carry you throughout your health hacker journey.

Now get outside, soak up some sunlight, and listen to some good-mood tunes to celebrate your SELF on this great day! You deserve it.

Summary:

- As of 2008, for the first time ever, the world's population was evenly split between urban and rural areas. Urbanization has continued, with more people now living in an urban setting than a rural setting.
- People's chronic disconnection with nature may cause them to underestimate nature's health benefits, and these forecasting errors may lead them to choose not to spend more time in nature.
- According to data from the US Centers for Disease Control and Prevention (CDC) National Health and Nutrition Examination Survey, nearly one in ten children has a Vitamin D deficiency.
- Forest bathing, or *Shinrin-yoku* in Japanese, is a real thing people do specifically for the benefits of time spent in nature—not physically bathing in any sort of liquid, but simply spending leisure time in the forest.
- Music is a free, boundless art form we can use to support the thoughts, feelings, and state we want to create.
- Listening to music out loud triggers the release of the hormones oxytocin (the love hormone) and serotonin (impacts our mood, sleep, and sex-drive).
- Personal electronic devices emit electromagnetic radiation (EMR), which a growing number of doctors and scientists warn may increase the risk of various diseases.
- Sustainable behavior change rarely happens without one thing—**finding joy.**
- Let your heart lead you and your joy carry you throughout your health hacker journey.

Action Items:

1. Follow the steps outlined earlier to experiment with spending more time in nature. Consider marking your calendar for going on a hike or simply taking a morning, afternoon, or evening walk outside. Ask yourself how you can get outside just a little bit more.

2. Experiment with new ways of optimizing your music experience.
    - How do you listen to music (e.g., CD in your car or music on your laptop, smartphone, or tablet)?
    - What type of music do you listen to and why?
    - When do you listen to music?
    - Do you use music to motivate, enhance, or bring joy to an activity? If so, which activities?

3. Add intentional music to your daily routines.
    - There are several great options for using music to support us during the day at night. I suggest trying out the artist Moby on Soundcloud, specifically his fifteen-minute, non-lyrical song titled "Live Forever." This song has brought more peace, understanding, and relaxation to me than any other song I've heard. Consider adding this song and a few others to your Evening Routine playlist on Soundcloud or Spotify.
    - **BONUS:** Listen to Moby's "Live Forever" while doing a relaxing activity, such as stretching, meditating, doing breathwork, or taking a warm shower or Epsom salt bath.

4. Protect Your Self. Do some research and consider purchasing radiation-blocking phone and laptop cases from SafeSleeve, unplugging your router at night, or grabbing a pair of Dr. Mercola's Blue Tube headphones.

5. Choose Joy. Consider choosing one activity to do this week that you truly enjoy. This can be anything. And it doesn't have to be related to your health. It just has to bring you happiness and joy.

NEXT STEPS

Thank you for taking the time to read *The Art of Health Hacking*. I am honored by your commitment to your health and hope that this book has provided you with some tools to make your health journey more fun, effortless, and successful.

If this book resonated with you and you're interested in learning more, join the conversation! We have some great free tools and a growing community of health hackers to support you in your quest to elevate your state. We also offer online challenges, group masterminds, and in-person workshops and events for you or your organization. And if you just want to stay in the loop, share your health hacking success stories, or ask some questions, that's great too!

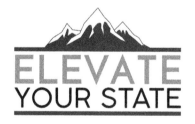

http://www.ElevateYourState.co
http://www.HealthHackerBook.com

Remember, health hacking is a process and a journey. And we, as health hackers, are called to continue developing the courage, willingness, and skill to elevate the quality of our life experience—one moment and day at a time.

ACKNOWLEDGEMENTS

Mom: You raised me with a special kind of love any child would dream of. And you were one of my original inspirations for becoming passionate about health! Without your love, presence, and positivity, I may not have persevered to finish this book.

Dad: You're an inspiration to me. You always have been. You taught me a job worth doing is worth doing well, which helped fuel my commitment to finishing this book strong. I also find it fitting you wrote your first book, *Check The Oil*, about antique gas pumps at about the same age I wrote this book—twenty-nine. Without your entrepreneurial spirit and passion for hard work and creativity, this book would not have been possible.

I am so grateful for everything you two have done for me in my life.

To my early readers and supporters of the crowdfunding campaign for this book, especially Brian Appleton, Michael Caira, Lee Constantine, Amanda Gyuran, Chris James, Skip Kelly, Wesley King, Thaddeus Own, Joel Sprechman, April Stickelman, Rae Swanson, and Guy Vincent: Thank you. Your support and excitement for me throughout this book writing process kept me motivated to deliver a high-quality finished product. Thank you for believing in me, sharing your stories, and having fun as we build a powerful health hacking community!

To all the health leaders who I interviewed for this book, especially Dave Asprey, Ben Greenfield, Kirstin Keilty, Garrett Salpeter, Daniel Schmachtenberger, Tony Stubblebine, and JJ Virgin, thank you for your contribution to the personal health empowerment movement and for taking the time to share your message with me and this health hacking community.

To my editors, Ashley Thoreson and Sara Stibitz:

Thank you so much for your hard work on this project, Ashley. This book wouldn't even be readable if it weren't for you. You rocked it. And you're my sister, so it's been pretty cool for us to work together like this.

Sara, your support and guidance early on in the editing process was quite impactful. You helped me own my story and my unique voice in a way I never thought possible. Thank you for believing in me as an author whose first (and possibly only) book always felt a bit rough around the edges. I'm thankful to call you a great friend for life.

To my friends and colleagues working in and around the health care, healing, and health optimization communities, Dr. Bill Appelgate, Dr. Anthony Balduzzi, Dr. Katherine Zagone, Kirstin Keilty, and the emergency responders who rushed me to the ER for dehydration while writing this book: Thank you for your commitment to your work. Showing up every day to help bring a higher level of health and quality of life for all is moving mountains. We all have a unique path or calling that adds value to the world. And in one way or another, through our relationships, you each helped me find mine.

And for every other friend, family member, and colleague I've built a relationship with before and during this book writing process: I am thankful for you. I appreciate your friendship, guidance, and commitment to living an awesome life. It's an honor to know you. Let's continue having fun and supporting each other in this health hacker journey as we make a major impact on the world.

ABOUT THE AUTHOR

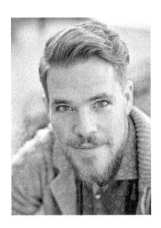

TJ ANDERSON is a self-proclaimed "health hacker," health care entrepreneur, speaker, and founder of Elevate Your State, a growing community of health-conscious consumers. Specializing in health coaching for behavior change and personal health empowerment, he has consulted for employers, medical groups, and several innovative health care organizations—Live Healthy Iowa, the Clinical Health Coach, and Breakthrough Physical Therapy Marketing—all using a unique approach to make a meaningful impact on the future of health care. TJ is dedicated to helping high-performing entrepreneurs, business professionals, CEO's, and parents everywhere to merge the fundamentals with the cutting edge to stay on top of their health game. You can find him online at http://www.ThisIsTJ.com or http://www.ElevateYourState.co.

RESOURCES

Products

SafeSleeve Cases: https://www.safesleevecases.com

Bulletproof: https://www.bulletproof.com

MyIntent Project: https://www.myintent.org

EnviroMedica (Ancient Minerals Magnesium Bath Flakes): https://www.enviromedica.com

Four Sigmatic (Reishi Mushrooms, Lions Mane for brain boost, Reishi for calming state, and Mushroom Coffee for a big brain and body boost): https://us.foursigmatic.com

EAD Labs (BioCBD+'s Total Body Care Capsules, Muscle and Joint Relief CBD Oil): https://eadlabs.com

Thrive pure CBD vape cartridge by VapeBright: https://www.vapebright.org/product/thrive

Dr. Mercola's Blue Tube Headphones: http://products.mercola.com/blue-tube-headset

Supplements

TJ's Favorite Supplements: http://www.ThisisTJ.com/FavoriteSupplements

Cannabidiol (CBD): https://www.biocbdplus.com

Neurohacker Collective (Qualia): http://neurohacker.com

Natural Stacks (MagTech Magnesium supplement and Branched Chain Amino Acids, BCAAs): https://www.naturalstacks.com

ONNIT (New MOOD Daily Stress Formula): https://www.onnit.com

Tools

Trigger Point Foam Roller: https://www.tptherapy.com

MyoBuddy Massager Pro: https://www.myobuddy.com

The Oh Ball Premium Massage Ball Roller: https://www.theohball.com

The Rolflex: https://irolflex.com

The Balsaq: https://www.indiegogo.com/projects/balsaq-ultimate-mobility-solution-fitness-health#

The Wave Tool: http://www.wavetools.net

Services

WellnessFX (Advanced Heart Health Test): https://www.wellnessfx.com

Holistic Health International (Dr. Amy Yasko, Health Tests): http://HolisticHeal.com

Raw DNA Sequencing: www.23andme.com

Sterling's App: https://MTHFRsupport.com

Genetic Genie: http://geneticgenie.org

LiveWello: https://livewello.com

SpectraCell Micronutrient Test (MNT): https://www.spectracell.com

HeartMath's Inner Health App and Device: https://www.heartmath.com

Websites, Blogs, & Podcasts

Ben Greenfield: https://BenGreenfieldFitness.com

NeuFit: https://www.neu.fit

Bulletproof: https://blog.bulletproof.com

Bulletproof Diet Roadmap Infographic: https://blog.bulletproof.com/wp-content/uploads/2016/02/BulletproofRoadmap_Rebrand_outlined.pdf

Wim Hof Method: https://WimHofMethod.com

Dr. Andrew Rostenberg: http://www.beyondmthfr.com

Dr. Amy Yasko: http://www.dramyyasko.com

Katherine M. Zagone, Naturopathic Doctor: http://theholisticfertilitymethod.com

American Osteopathic Association: http://www.osteopathic.org

American Association of Naturopathic Physicians: http://www.naturopathic. org

American Chiropractic Association: https://www.acatoday.org

American Physical Therapy Association: https://www.apta.org

Institute for Functional Medicine: https://www.ifm.org

Medi-Share: https://mychristiancare.org

JJ Virgin Sugar Impact Quiz: http://virgindietcommunity.com/sidresources/ wp-content/uploads/2014/10/SUGAR-IMPACT-QUIZ.pdf

Brain.fm: https://www.brain.fm

Wholetones: https://wholetones.com

Calm.com: https://www.calm.com

YouTube: https://www.youtube.com

Spotify: https://www.spotify.com

Sound Cloud: https://soundcloud.com

Health Coaching & Training

Iowa Chronic Care Consortium: http://iowaccc.com

Healthy for Life University: https://healthyforlifeusa.com/pages/healthy-for-life-u

Clinical Health Coach: http://clinicalhealthcoach.com

Nudge: https://nudgecoach.com

Coach.Me: https://www.coach.me

Twine: https://www.twinehealth.com

Books

The Patient Will See You Now by Eric Topol

The Biology of Belief—10th Anniversary Edition by Bruce Lipton

Self-Compassion: The Proven Power of Being Kind to Yourself by Kristin Neff

The Presence Process by Michael Brown

Thought as Passion by Frank Visser

Integral Christianity: The Spirit's Call to Evolve by Paul R. Smith

Secrets of the Millionaire Mind by T. Harv Ecker

Alone Together: Why We Expect More from Technology and Less from Each Other by Sherry Turkle

Cholesterol Clarity: What the HDL is Wrong with My Numbers by Jimmy Moore and Eric C. Westman

The Paleo Cardiologist: The Natural Way to Heart Health by Jack Wolfson

Grain Brain: The Surprising Truth about Wheat, Carbs, and Sugar—Your Brain's Silent Killers by Dr. David Perlmutter

The Bulletproof Diet by Dave Asprey

The Nature Fix: Why Nature Makes us Happier, Healthier, and More Creative by Florence Williams

The Dorito Effect: The Surprising Truth About Food and Flavor by Mark Schatzker

The Sugar Impact Diet by JJ Virgin

Last Child in the Woods by Richard Louv

NOTES

How to Use This Book

Leonardo da Vinci: Advameg Inc. "Leonardo Da Vinci Biography." *Encyclopedia of World Biography*. Accessed October 28, 2017. http://www.notablebiographies.com/Ki-Lo/Leonardo-da-Vinci.html.

Da Vinci taught himself about human anatomy: Jones, "Leonardo Da Vinci."

Meta-analysis of studies on body weight around the world: Ng et al., "Global, Regional, and National Prevalence."

Life expectancy and health care spending: Uberti, "Cost of Health Care by Country," using OECD Health Data 2009 (data gathered in 2007).

Fifty thousand health apps available: Zhang and Koch, "Mobile Health Apps in Sweden."

Five-Act Structure: Ray, Rebecca. "The Five Act Play (Dramatic Structure)." *Storyboard That*. Accessed October 29, 2017. http://www.storyboardthat.com/articles/e/five-act-structure/.

Da Vinci, "I have been impressed with the urgency of doing": BrainyQuote, "Leonardo Da Vinci Quotes," 2017, https://www.brainyquote.com/quotes/quotes/l/leonardoda120052.html.

ACT 1

Chapter 1: Goodbye, Sick-Care; Hello, Self-Care

Buckminster Fuller, "You never change things by fighting the existing reality": Goodreads Inc., 2017, https://www.goodreads.com/quotes/13119-you-never-change-things-by-fighting-the-existing-reality-to/.

Dr. Bill Appelgate, "Much of health care is organized and delivered": The Clinical Health Coach Training Online, Iowa Chronic Care Consortium, 2017, http://clinicalhealthcoach.com/online-overview/.

Defintion of health care: Merriam-Webster's Online Dictionary, Definition of Health Care, 2017, https://www.merriam-webster.com/dictionary/health%20care.

Biggest health care problem, acute versus chronic disease: Gerteis et al., *Multiple Chronic Conditions*, 1.

"Every system is perfectly designed": Carr, "Editor's Notebook."

Ben Greenfield, "The emergency room is a good place to go if": Ben Greenfield, interview by TJ Anderson, San Diego, CA, October 20, 2015.

A third of US health care spending is wasted: Smith et al., *Best Care at Lower Cost*, 104.

$750 billion to $760 billion wasted on unnecessary services: IOM, *The Healthcare Imperative*, 2.

The traditional health care system is bankrupting our country: IOM, *The Healthcare Imperative*, 13.

Precision Medicine Initiative: "Fact Sheet: President Obama's Precision Medicine Initiative," The White House, Office of the Press Secretary, January 30, 2015, https://obamawhitehouse.archives.gov/the-press-office/2015/01/30/fact-sheet-president-obama-s-precision-medicine-initiative.

Eric Topol, "The first time I had an ECG emailed to me by a patient": Topol, *The Patient Will See You Now*, 6.

Craig Venter, HLI, sequencing the human genome, "If we can predict at birth": Human Longevity Inc., "Introducing Human Longevity Inc. Health Nucleus," *YouTube* video, 04:16, Posted October 27, 2015, https://www.youtube.com/watch?v=QwS-b-stG7o.

Peter Diamandis, The Health Nucleus, "make healthcare predictive and preventative," "As we get older, our stem cell population": Ferriss, "Peter Diamandis."

Dr. Bill Applegate, "The power of health coaching is to do three things": The Clinical Health Coach Training Online, Iowa Chronic Care Consortium, 2017, http://clinicalhealthcoach.com/online-overview/.

80–80–80 Rule: The Clinical Health Coach Training Online, Iowa Chronic Care Consortium, 2017, http://clinicalhealthcoach.com/online-overview/.

Pathogenesis, origin and treatment of disease: Merriam-Webster's Online Dictionary, Definition of Pathogenesis, 2017, https://www.merriam-webster.com/dictionary/pathogenesis.

Antonovsky, Salutogenesis: Mittelmark and Bauer, "Chapter 2: The Meanings of Salutogenesis," 7.

Salutogenesis, "salus" and "genesis," the origin and creation of health: "Salutogenesis," *Wikipedia*, last modified November 6, 2017, https://en.wikipedia.org/wiki/Salutogenesis.

Definition of Self-Care: WHO, *The Role of the Pharmacist*, 2.

Chapter 2: Beyond The Physical

Einstein, "We can't solve problems": BrainyQuote, "Albert Einstein Quotes," 2017, https://www.brainyquote.com/quotes/quotes/a/alberteins385842.html.

Dr. Shelton quote, Etymology of the word health: Bidwell, Victoria. "The Etymology of the Word 'Health'" *Get Well Stay Well America.* Accessed October 29, 2017. http://www.getwellstaywellamerica.com/EnergyEnhancers/etymologyHealth.htm.

WHO definition of "Health": "Constitution of WHO Principles," World Health Organization, 2017, http://www.who.int/about/mission/en/.

Living Proof Institute, Figure 1 Image: Reprinted with permission from The Living Proof Institute, 2017, https://thelivingproofinstitute.com/about/.

Lipton, The Biology of Belief, changes in genetic expression and disease: Lipton, *The Biology of Belief.*

Lipton, "Our health is not controlled by genetics," the subconscious mind controls 95 percent of our lives, "The function of the mind is to create coherence": Forston, *Embrace, Release, Heal*, 160.

Data suggest 90 to 95 percent of cancer: Anand et al., "Cancer is a Preventable Disease," 2097.

Chapter 3: What's Your Story?

Aristotle, "Educating the mind": Goodreads Inc., 2017, https://www. goodreads.com/quotes/95080-educating-the-mind-without-educating-the-heart-is-no-education.

Kristin Neff, "The only way to truly have compassion for yourself": Neff, *Self-Compassion*, 19.

Da Vinci, the heart, not the liver, was central to the blood system: Jones, "Leonardo Da Vinci."

4 Levels of Truth Telling: Jesse Elder, "4 Levels of Truth Telling," Phil Drolet's World Class Accelerator Mastermind, March 2014.

Kristin Neff, Letter-Writing Exercise: Kristin Neff, "Exercise 3: Exploring Self-Compassion through Writing," *Self-Compassion*, 2017, http://self-compassion. org/exercise-3-exploring-self-compassion-writing/.

ACT 2
Chapter 4: Hacking and Tracking Change Everything

Einstein, "Not everything that counts can be counted…": Toye, "'Not Everything that can be Counted.'"

Garrett Salpeter, NeuFit: Garrett Salpeter (NeuFit), phone interview and email communication with author, October 10, 2017.

Gary Wolf, TEDx Cannes, "The self is our operating center," "I got up this morning," "Now we know that new tools": Wolf, "The Quantified Self."

Wearables market will grow almost threefold by 2019: "Wearables Market to be Worth $25 Billion by 2019," *CSS Insight*, 2017, http://www.ccsinsight.com/ press/company-news/2332-wearables-market-to-be-worth-25-billion-by-2019-reveals-ccs-insight/.

Biohacking documentary episode of SHIFT: Steve Adams and Sean Horlor, "SHIFT: Biohacking Documentary," *Nootka St. Film Company*. YouTube video, 12:52. Posted May 21, 2015. https://www.youtube.com/ watch?v=B75zyFDVPGc.

Dr. Mark Ashton Smith, biohacking movement, "Biohacking has joined forces": Smith, "Introduction to Self Quantification."

Dave Asprey, Bulletproof, "I lost 100 pounds," "Carve your own path": Dave Asprey (founder and CEO of Bulletproof), Skype video interview by author, April 8, 2015.

Chapter 5: What is Health Hacking?

Emma Hill, "Every patient is an expert": Hill, "Smart Patients," 141.

Definition of health literacy: U.S. Department of Health and Human Services. *Quick Guide to Health Literacy*, 2.1.

Chapter 6: From Health Coaching to Self Coaching: It Starts With A Question

Cheryl James, "Change is not an event": BrainyQuote, "Cheryl James Quotes," 2017, https://www.brainyquote.com/quotes/quotes/c/cheryljame421502.html.

Jim Kwik, "Your mind is always eavesdropping": Dave Asprey, "Jim Kwik: Speed Reading, Memory, & Superlearning—Episode #189," Transcript and *Bulletproof Radio* video, Posted January 16, 2015, 32:17, https://blog.bulletproof.com/jim-kwik-speed-reading-memory-superlearning-189/.

Twine Health, April 2016 survey: Emily Wolfe, "Consumer Survey: The State of Health Coaching in 2016," *Twine Health*, April 25, 2016, https://www.twinehealth.com/blog/consumer-survey-the-state-of-health-coaching-in-2016/.

Dr. Roger Jahnke, "People with medical degrees": Fuscaldo, "Do You Need a Health Coach."

The Transtheoretical Model of Behavior Change: "The Transtheoretical Model," Pro-Change Behavior Systems Inc., 2017, https://www.prochange.com/transtheoretical-model-of-behavior-change; and Prochaska et al., "In Search of How People Change."

Motivational Interviewing and Defining O.A.R.S: Miller and Rollnick, *Motivational Interviewing*, 62–73.

ACT 3
Chapter 7: Create Clarity

Michael Brown, "During this journey": Brown, *The Presence Process*, 30.

Chapter 8: You're Not Alone: The Power of God
and Close Relationships

Wayne Dyer, "You are a creature of divine love": AZquotes, http://www.azquotes.com/quote/857139.

Ken Wilber, Integral Theory, "The word integral": Wilber, "Foreword," xii.

Paul Smith, Jesus as a mystic, "Mystical experience is available to everyone": Smith, *Integral Christianity*, 143-144.

Paul Smith, "For most of my life I have believed": Smith, *Integral Christianity*, 288–289.

Paul Smith, two types of prayer: Smith, *Integral Christianity*, 294–299.

Circling: The Integral Center, "What is Circling," 2017, http://integralcenter.org/circling/.

Chapter 9: Define Your Why

Wayne Dyer, "When you change the way you look at things": Fearless Soul, "If You Change the Way You Look at Things, the Things You Look at Change," June 22, 2016, https://iamfearlesssoul.com/if-you-change-the-way-you-look-at-things-the-things-you-look-at-change/.

Ecker, "The roots create the fruit": Ecker, *Millionaire Mind*, 12, 31.

Ecker, financial blueprint: Ecker, *Millionaire Mind*, 2–7.

Michael Brown, allow our intention to meet our attention: Brown, *The Presence Process*.

ACT 4
Chapter 10: Take a Break, Take a Breath

Mister Rogers, "In times of stress, the best thing we can do": Goodreads Inc., Fred Rogers from *The World According to Mister Rogers*, 2017, https://www.goodreads.com/quotes/309644-in-times-of-stress-the-best-thing-we-can-do/.

APA 2010 Stress in America survey, 44 percent of adults in the United States report their level of stress has increased: Clay, "Stressed in America," 60.

APA 2017 Stress in America survey, "unplugging" and taking a "digital detox" important for mental health: APA, *Stress in America*, 3.

APA 2017 Stress in America survey, constantly checking email, texts, and social media report higher levels of stress: APA, *Stress in America*, 1.

Sherry Turkle, "The self shaped in a world of rapid response": Turkle, *Alone Together*, 166.

Sherry Turkle, virtual identity: Turkle, *Alone Together*, 256.

Dr. Mark Hyman, the medical definition of stress: Hyman, "5 Ways to Never Be Stressed Again."

Wim Hof Method and Warning, "The breathing exercise": "Practice the Wim Hof Method," *Wim Hof Method*, Accessed November 4, 2017. https://www.wimhofmethod.com/practice-the-method.

John C. Lilly, sensory deprivation tanks: Caruso, *Revolutionize Your Corporate Life*, 127.

Hot and cold showers: Dale, "Hot or Cold?"

Chapter 11: Measure What Matters

Andrew Rostenberg, "Not only are our genes powerful": Andrew Rostenberg, *Beyond MTHFR*, 2016, http://www.BeyondMTHFR.com.

Ketogenic diet, epilepsy treatment: "What is the Ketogenic Diet," The Charlie Foundation, 2017, https://www.charliefoundation.org/explore-ketogenic-diet/explore-1/introducing-the-diet.

Jimmy Moore and Dr. Eric Westman, Cholesterol Clarity: Moore and Westman, *Cholesterol Clarity*.

Cardiovascular disease and size and density of LDL particles: "Advanced Heart Health." *WellnessFX*. 2017. https://www.wellnessfx.com/advanced-heart-health; "Cholesterol is not Evil but High Lp(a) is a Killer." *The Drs. Wolfson*. May 4, 2017. https://www.thedrswolfson.com/how-to-lower-lpa/; and Saleheen et al., "Apolipoprotein(a) Isoform Size."

Dr. Amy Yasko, the methylation cycle: "The Methylation Cycle," Dr. Amy Yasko, Holistic Health International, 2017, http://www.dramyyasko.com/our-unique-approach/methylation-cycle/.

Dr. Mercola, "While scientists refer to Vitamin D as a vitamin": "Vitamin D Resource Page," Dr. Joseph Mercola, 2017, http://www.mercola.com/article/vitamin-d-resources.htm/.

Kirstin Keilty, "Nutrition is a concert": Kirstin Keilty, MS, CNS (Clinical Consultant at SpectraCell Laboratories), phone interview by author, November 29, 2016.

HeartMath and Heart Rate Variability (HRV): HeartMath Inc. "The Science of HeartMath," 2017, https://www.heartmath.com/science/.

Dave Asprey on HRV training, "When you use this little game": Dave Asprey (founder and CEO of Bulletproof), Skype video interview by author, April 8, 2015.

Chapter 12: How to Build Your Health Care Team

Dr. Mark Hyman, "Functional medicine is about causes, not symptoms": Jeremy Miller, "20 Quotes from the Functional Medicine Institute." *The Healthy Choice*, January 27, 2014, https://healthychoicenews.wordpress.com/2014/01/27/20-quotes-from-the-functional-medicine-institute/.

IFM, Functional Medicine model definition: "Functional Medicine," The Institute for Functional Medicine, 2017, https://www.ifm.org/functional-medicine/.

Ahn et al., Reductionism, "A young immunocompromised man" and "Rather than dividing a complex problem": Ahn et al., "The Limits of Reductionism," 709.

Ahn et al., Integrative Approach, "In clinical medicine, complex, chronic diseases": Ahn et al., "The Clinical Applications of a Systems Approach," 957.

DOs are trained in a whole-person approach: "What is a DO?", American Osteopathic Association (AOA), 2017, http://www.osteopathic.org/osteopathic-health/about-dos/what-is-a-do/Pages/default.aspx.

NDs combine the wisdom of nature with the rigors of modern-day science: "What is a Naturopathic Doctor?" American Academy of Naturopathic Physicians (AANP), 2017, http://www.naturopathic.org/content.asp?contentid=60.

Millions of Americans experiencing back pain: Jensen et al., "Magnetic Resonance Imaging," 69.

Ben Greenfield, building your health care team, "There are three things to look at": Ben Greenfield, interview by author, San Diego, CA, October 20, 2015.

Asking good questions before selecting your doctor of choice: "Questions for Functional Medicine Practitioners," The Institute for Functional Medicine, 2014, https://p.widencdn.net/iymmsf/Questions-For-Functional-Medicine-Practitioners.

ACT 5
Chapter 13: The Paradox of Goals

Eisenhower, "In preparing for battle": BrainyQuote, "Dwight D. Eisenhower Quotes," 2017, https://www.brainyquote.com/quotes/quotes/d/dwightdei164720.html.

Five Stages of Change, Reviewed: "The Transtheoretical Model," Pro-Change Behavior Systems Inc., 2017, https://www.prochange.com/transtheoretical-model-of-behavior-change.

Rollnick, Mason, and Butler, Health Behavior Change, "If a change feels important to you," importance and confidence: Rollnick et al., *Health Behavior Change*, 17–18.

Conversation Flow Model: *The Clinical Health Coach Training Online*, Iowa Chronic Care Consortium, 2017, http://clinicalhealthcoach.com/online-overview/.

James Clear, three reasons to focus on systems instead of goals: Clear, "Forget about Setting Goals."

S.M.A.R.T. goals: *The Clinical Health Coach Training Online*, Iowa Chronic Care Consortium, 2017, http://clinicalhealthcoach.com/online-overview/.

Tony Stubblebine, experimentation and momentum: Tony Stubblebine, Skype video interview by author, April 29, 2016.

James Clear, "Feedback loops are important for building good systems": Clear, "Forget about Setting Goals."

Chapter 14: Your Daily Routine

Edison, "The doctor of the future": Isaak and Siow, "The Evolution of Nutrition Research," Abstract.

Dr. David Perlmutter, Grain Brain, impact of nutrition on the brain: Perlmutter, *Grain Brain.*

Samantha Olson, 2,200 flavor chemicals, "A once simple system of nutritional nourishment": Olson, "The Food Industry."

Mark Schatzker, The Dorito Effect, "We could live in a world where food tastes very good": Olson, "The Food Industry."

20 percent tax on sugary drinks: WHO, *Fiscal Policies,* 24.

JJ Virgin, The Sugar Impact Diet, Taper, Transition, and Transform: Virgin, *The Sugar Impact Diet,* xxiii.

JJ Virgin, "If you go cold turkey on sugar": JJ Virgin, Skype video interview with author, August 17, 2015.

Your brain lags behind your stomach: Christa Miller, "How Long Does It Take Your Brain to Register That the Stomach is Full," Livestrong.com, July 18, 2017, https://www.livestrong.com/article/480254-how-long-does-it-take-your-brain-to-register-that-the-stomach-is-full/.

Benefits of short-term, intermittent fasting: Collier, "Intermittent Fasting."

Nootropics, "smart drugs": What are "Nootropics," *Smart Drug Smarts,* 2017, https://smartdrugsmarts.com/faq/nootropics/.

Qualia: "Formulation," *Neurohacker Collective,* 2017, formulation; and "Applied Neuropsychopharmacology," *Neurohacker Collective,* 2017, http://neurohacker.com/applied/.

Qualia is not for everyone, should not be taken by people on MAO inhibitors, SSRIs, or any other psychiatric medicines: "Is it safe? Who is it safe for?" *Neurohacker Collective,* 2016, https://neurohacker.zendesk.com/hc/en-us/articles/224362868-Is-it-safe-Who-is-it-safe-for-/.

Daniel Schmachtenberger, "We affect and are affected by our environment": Daniel Schmachtenberger (Neurohacker Collective), Skype video interview by author, Video call, September 1, 2016.

Workouts that involve short bursts of high heart rate movement: Ramos et al., "The Impact of High-Intensity Interval Training."

H.I.I.T. workouts may result in reduced enjoyment of over time: Foster et al., "The Effects of High Intensity Interval Training," 749-751.

Gene Tunney, "Exercise should be regarded as a tribute": Whitney Hopler, "Motivational Quotes on Fitness and Wellness." *Center for the Advancement of Well-Being.* October 17, 2017. https://wellbeing.gmu.edu/articles/11192/.

Sunlight exposure signals your hypothalamus: "The Hypothalamus, Pituitary and Pineal Glands," Epidemic Answers, 2014. https://epidemicanswers.org/reference-library/hormones/hypothalamus-pituitary-pineal/.

Blue light disrupts melatonin production: Tosini et al., "Effects of Blue Light," 65.

Oura ring, more accurate readings than if worn on your wrist: Kinnunen, "Sleep Lab Validation," 5.

Ben Greenfield, 80/20 principle, "Set up a system where": Ben Greenfield, interview by author, San Diego, CA, October 20, 2015.

JJ Virgin, journaling as best health hack: JJ Virgin, Skype video interview by author, August 17, 2015.

Chapter 15: Nature, Music, and Enjoying the Ride

Shakespeare, "One touch of nature": BrainyQuote, "William Shakespeare Quotes," 2017, https://www.brainyquote.com/quotes/quotes/w/williamsha106907.html.

APA 2017 Stress in America survey: APA, *Stress in America*, 3.

Nisbet and Zelenski, forecasting errors: Nisbet and Zelenski, "Underestimating Nearby Nature."

Urbanization, world's urban versus rural population as of 2008: "Human Population: Urbanization," *Population Reference Bureau*, 2016, http://www.prb.org/Publications/Lesson-Plans/HumanPopulation/Urbanization.aspx/.

Degree of urbanization as of 2017: "Urbanization by Continent 2017," *Statista*, 2017, https://www.statista.com/statistics/270860/urbanization-by-continent/.

Nearly one in ten, 7.6 million, children Vitamin D deficient; 50.8 million children Vitamin D insufficient: Kumar et al., "Prevalence and Associations," e365.

Florence Williams, The Nature Fix, "Yet we think of nature as a luxury": Williams, *The Nature Fix*, 12.

Forest bathing, "The Japanese go crazy for this practice": Williams, *The Nature Fix*, 17–18.

Japanese forests cover 68 percent of the country's landmass, $4 million in forest-bathing research, Forest Therapy trails: Williams, *The Nature Fix*, 19.

Viewing and walking in Japanese forest sites results in better moods, lower anxiety, changes in physiological states: Williams, *The Nature Fix*, 23.

Physiological data collected at Japanese forest sites: Lee et al., "Nature Therapy," 329–334.

Nature-Deficit Disorder: Louv, *Last Child in the Woods*.

Dr. Daniel Levitin, music and the brain: Levitin, *This Is Your Brain On Music*.

Levitin, Sonos, and Apple research study data; the role of music in our homes and lives: Titlow, "How Music Changes Your Behavior;" "Can Music Out Loud Change the Way we Connect at Home?" February 9, 2016. http://musicmakesithome.com/post/138963081132/what-is-going-on.

Dr. Daniel Levitin, "Nexus of intimacy and togetherness," there's a neurochemical basis for findings, "We find from studies": Titlow, "How Music Changes Your Behavior."

SafeSleeve, Electromagnetic Radiation: https://www.safesleevecases.com/pages/emfinfo/.

Dr. Mercola's Blue Tube Headphones: http://products.mercola.com/blue-tube-headset/.

BIBLIOGRAPHY

Ahn, Andrew C., Muneesh Tewari, Chi-Sang Poon, and Russell S. Phillips. "The Limits of Reductionism in Medicine: Could Systems Biology Offer an Alternative?" *Public Library of Science (PLOS) Medicine* 3, issue 6 (June 2006): 709–713. doi: 10.1371/journal.pmed.0030208.

———."The Clinical Applications of a Systems Approach." *Public Library of Science (PLOS) Medicine* 3, issue 7 (July 2006): 956–960. doi: 10.1371/journal.pmed.0030209.

American Psychological Association (APA). *Stress in America: Coping with Change, Part 2*. Stress in America Survey. 10th ed. February 23, 2017. https://www.apa.org/news/press/releases/stress/2017/technology-social-media.PDF.

Anand, Preetha, Ajaikumar B. Kunnumakara, Chitra Sundaram, Kuzhuvelil B. Harikumar, Sheeja T. Tharakan, Oiki S. Lai, Bokyung Sung, and Bharat B. Aggarwal. "Cancer is a Preventable Disease that Requires Major Lifestyle Changes." *Pharmaceutical Research* 25, no. 9 (Sept 2008): 2097–2116. doi: 10.1007/s11095-008-9661-9.

Appelgate, William. "Promoting Health, Preventing Disease, and Prompting Population Progress." In *The Role of Telehealth in an Evolving Health Care Environment, The Health Care Continuum, Institute of Medicine Workshop Summary*, Tracy A. Lustig, 43–46. Washington, D.C.: The National Academies Press, 2012. https://www.ncbi.nlm.nih.gov/books/NBK207138/.

Brown, Michael. *The Presence Process.* Vancouver: Namaste Publishing, 2010.

Burke, Jennifer. "GOP Candidates Dive into the True Cost Drivers in Our Economy." *Business Wire.* October 29, 2015. http://www.businesswire.com/news/home/20151029005828/en/GOP-Candidates-Dive-True-Cost-Drivers-Economy.

Carr, Susan. "Editor's Notebook: A Quotation with a Life of Its Own." *Patient Safety and Quality Healthcare.* July/August 2008. https://www.psqh.com/analysis/editor-s-notebook-a-quotation-with-a-life-of-its-own/.

Caruso, Peggy. *Revolutionize Your Corporate Life- A Simple Guide to Leadership, Balance and Success in Your Business.* New York: Morgan James Publishing, 2017.

Clark, Alan. *The Sociology of Healthcare.* 2nd ed. New York: Routledge, 2010.

Clay, R.A. "Stressed in America." *Monitor on Psychology* 42, no. 1 (Jan 2011): 60 (print version). http://www.apa.org/monitor/2011/01/stressed-america.aspx/.

Clear, James. "Forget about Setting Goals. Focus on This Instead." *James Clear.* 2017. https://jamesclear.com/goals-systems.

Collier, Roger. "Intermittent Fasting: The Science of Going Without." *Canadian Medical Association Journal* 185, no. 9 (June 2013): 363–364. doi:10.1503/cmaj.109-4451.

Dale, Heather. "Hot or Cold? The Benefits of Both Kinds of Showers." *Popsugar.* November 3, 2017. https://www.popsugar.com/fitness/Cold-Showers-vs-Hot-Showers-Health-Benefits-Both-15021710/.

Ecker, T. Harv. *Secrets of the Millionaire Mind.* New York: Harper Collins Publishers, 2005.

Ferriss, Tim. "Peter Diamandis on Disrupting the Education System, The Future of Healthcare, and Building a Billion-Dollar Business." *The Tim Ferriss Show.* Podcast Audio. July 17, 2015. http://tim.blog/2015/07/17/peter-diamandis-on-the-education-system/.

Forston, Leigh. *Embrace, Release, Heal: An Empowering Guide to Talking About, Thinking About, and Treating Cancer.* Boulder: Sounds True Inc., 2011.

Foster, Carl, Courtney V. Farland, Flavia Guidotti, Michelle Harbin, Brianna Roberts, Jeff Schuette, Andrew Tuuri, Scott T. Doberstein, and John P. Porcari. "The Effects of High Intensity Interval Training vs. Steady State Training on Aerobic and Anaerobic Capacity." *Journal of Sports Science and Medicine* 14, issue 4 (Dec 2015): 747-755. https://www.ncbi.nlm. nih.gov/pmc/articles/PMC4657417/.

Fuscaldo, Donna. "Do You Need a Health Coach." *Fox Business.com.* December 13, 2011. http://www.foxbusiness.com/features/2011/12/13/do-need-health-coach.html/.

Gerteis, Jessie, David Izrael, Deborah Deitz, Lisa LeRoy, Richard Ricciardi, Therese Miller, and Jayasree Basu. *Multiple Chronic Conditions Chartbook: 2010 Medical Expenditure Panel Survey Data.* Rockville, MD: Agency for Healthcare Research and Quality, April 2014, 1-45. https://www. ahrq.gov/sites/default/files/wysiwyg/professionals/prevention-chronic-care/decision/mcc/mccchartbook.pdf.

Hill, Emma. "Smart Patients." *The Lancet Oncology* 15, no. 2 (Feb 2014): 140–141. doi: http://dx.doi.org/10.1016/S1470-2045(14)70044-0.

Hyman, Mark. "5 Ways to Never Be Stressed Again." *Huffington Post (The Blog).* Last modified July 6, 2013. https://www.huffingtonpost.com/dr-mark-hyman/stress-tips_b_3178949.html/.

Institute of Medicine (IOM). *The Healthcare Imperative: Lowering Costs and Improving Outcomes: Workshop Series Summary, Learning Health System Series.* Washington, D.C.: The National Academies Press, 2010.

Isaak, Cara K., and Yaw L. Siow. "The Evolution of Nutrition Research." *Canadian Journal of Physiology and Pharmacology* 91, issue 4 (April 2013): 254–267.

Jensen Maureen C., Michael N. Brant-Zawadzki, Nancy Obuchowski, Michael T. Modic, Dennis Malkasian, and Jeffrey S. Ross. "Magnetic Resonance Imaging of the Lumbar Spine in People Without Back Pain." *New England Journal of Medicine* 331, no. 2 (July 1994): 69–73.

Jones, Roger. "Leonardo Da Vinci: Anatomist." *The British Journal of General Practice* 62, issue 599 (2012): 319. doi: 10.3399/bjgp12X649241.

Kinnunen, Hannu. "Sleep Lab Validation of a Wellness Ring in Detecting Sleep Patterns Based on Photoplethysmogram, Actigraphy and Body Temperature." *OURA Ring* (Feb 2016): 1–6. https://ouraring.com/wp-content/uploads/2017/08/Validity-of-the-OURA-Ring-in-determining-Sleep-Quantity-and-Quality-2016.pdf.

Kumar, Juhi, Paul Muntner, Frederick J. Kaskel, Susan M. Hailpern, and Michal L. Melamed. "Prevalence and Associations of 25-Hydroxyvitamin D Deficiency in US Children: NHANES 2001–2004." *Pediatrics* 124 no. 3 (Sept 2009): e362–e370. doi:10.1542/peds.2009-0051.

Lee, Juyoung, Qing Li, Liisa Tyrvainen, Yuko Tsunetsugu, Bum-Jin Park, Takahide Kagawa, and Yoshifumi Miyazaki. "Nature Therapy and Preventive Medicine." *In Public Health—Social and Behavioral Health*, edited by Jay Maddock, 325–350. In Tech, 2012. doi: 10.5772/37701.

Levitin, Daniel. *This Is Your Brain On Music*. New York: Plume, Penguin Inc., 2007.

Lipton, Bruce. *The Biology of Belief*. 10th Anniversary Edition. Carlsbad, CA: Hay House, 2016.

Louv, Richard. *Last Child in the Woods*. Chapel Hill: Algonquin Books of Chapel Hill, 2008.

Miller, William R., and Stephen Rollnick. *Motivational Interviewing: Helping People Change*. 3rd ed. New York: The Guilford Press, 2013.

Moore, Jimmy, and Eric C. Westman. *Cholesterol Clarity: What the HDL is Wrong with My Numbers*. Las Vegas: Victory Belt Publishing Inc., 2013.

Neff, Kristin. *Self-Compassion: The Proven Power of Being Kind to Yourself*. 2011. Reprint, New York: HarperCollins, 2015.

Ng, Marie, Tom Fleming, Margaret Robinson, Blake Thomson, Nicholas Graetz, Christopher Margono, Erin C. Mullany et al. "Global, Regional, and National Prevalence of Overweight and Obesity in Children and Adults during 1980–2013: A Systematic Analysis for the Global Burden of Disease Study 2013." *The Lancet* 384, issue 9945 (Aug 2014): 766–781. doi: 10.1016/S0140-6736(14)60460-8.

Nisbet, Elizabeth K., and John M. Zelenski. "Underestimating Nearby Nature: Affective Forecasting Errors Obscure the Happy Path to Sustainability."

Psychological Science 22, issue 9 (Aug 2011): 1101–1106. doi: 10.1177/0956797611418527.

Olson, Samantha. "The Food Industry Has Changed How Our Taste Buds Work." Medical Daily. July 14, 2015. http://www.medicaldaily.com/food-industry-has-changed-how-our-taste-buds-work-338098/.

Perlmutter, David. *Grain Brain: The Surprising Truth about Wheat, Carbs, and Sugar—Your Brain's Silent Killers.* New York: Little, Brown and Company, 2013.

Prochaska, James O., DiClemente, Carlo C., and Norcross, John C. "In Search of How People Change. Applications to Addictive Behaviors." *American Psychologist* 47, issue 9 (Sept 1992): 1102–1114. https://www.ncbi.nlm.nih.gov/pubmed/1329589.

Ramos, Joyce S., Lance C. Dalleck, Arnt Erik Tjonna, Kassia S. Beetham, and Jeff S. Coombes. "The Impact of High-Intensity Interval Training Versus Moderate-Intensity Continuous Training on Vascular Function: A Systemic Review and Meta-Analysis." *Sports Medicine* 45, issue 5, 679–692. doi: 10.1007/s40279-015-0321-z.

Rollnick, Stephen, Pip Mason, and Chris Butler. *Health Behavior Change.* 1st ed. London: Churchill Livingstone, Elsevier Limited, 1999.

Saleheen, Danish, Philip Haycock, Wei Zhao, Asif Rasheed, Adam Taleb, Atif Imran, Shahid Abbas et al. "Apolipoprotein(a) Isoform Size, Lipoprotein(a) Concentration, and Coronary Artery Disease: A Mendelia Randomisation Analysis." *Lancet Diabetes Endocrinology* 5 (Feb 2017): 524–533. http://dx.doi.org/10.1016/S2213-8587(17)30088-8.

Smith, Mark Ashton. "Introduction to Self Quantification and Biohacking." *IQ Mindware.* September 12, 2011. http://www.iqmindware.com/brain-train/mindhacks/introduction-brain-biohacking-dave-asprey/.

Smith, Mark, Robert Saunders, Leigh Stuckhardt, and J. Michael McGinnis, eds. *Best Care at Lower Cost: The Path to Continuously Learning Health Care in America.* Institute of Medicine. Washington, D.C.: National Academy of Sciences. doi: 10.17226/13444.

Smith, Paul R. *Integral Christianity: The Spirit's Call to Evolve.* 2011. Reprint, St. Paul, MN: Paragon House, 2012.

Titlow, John Paul. "How Music Changes Your Behavior At Home." *Fast Company*, February 10, 2016. https://www.fastcompany.com/3056554/how-music-changes-our-behavior-at-home.

Topol, Eric. *The Patient Will See You Now*. New York: Basic Books, 2015.

Tosini, Gianluca, Ian Ferguson, and Kazuo Tsubota. "Effects of Blue Light on the Circadian System and Eye Physiology." *Molecular Vision* 22 (Jan 2016): 61–72. http://www.molvis.org/molvis/v22/61/.

Toye, Francine. "'Not Everything that can be Counted Counts and Not Everything that Counts can be Counted' (attributed to Albert Einstein)." *British Journal of Pain* 9, issue 1 (Feb 2015): 7. https://www.ncbi.nlm.nih.gov/pmc/articles/PMC4616986/.

Turkle, Sherry. *Alone Together: Why We Expect More from Technology and Less from Each Other*. New York: Basic Books, 2012.

Uberti, Oliver. "Cost of Health Care by Country" Information Graphic. *National Geographic*, 2009. http://www.oliveruberti.com/infographics/ewpc0ylkniugxuu1gm8o0zy8f4jvft/.

U.S. Department of Health and Human Services. *Quick Guide to Health Literacy*. Washington, D.C.: Office of Disease Prevention and Health Promotion. Accessed November 2, 2017. https://health.gov/communication/literacy/quickguide/Quickguide.pdf/.

Virgin, JJ. *The Sugar Impact Diet*. New York: Grant Central Life & Style, 2014.

World Health Organization (WHO). *Fiscal Policies for Diet and Prevention of Noncommunicable Diseases: Technical Meeting Report*, May 5–6, 2015. Geneva: WHO, 2016. http://www.who.int/dietphysicalactivity/publications/fiscal-policies-diet-prevention/en/.

———. *The Role of the Pharmacist in Self-Care and Self-Medication*. Report of the 4th WHO Consultative Group on the Role of the Pharmacist. Geneva: WHO, 1998. http://apps.who.int/medicinedocs/en/d/Jwhozip32e/3.1.html/.

Wilber, Ken. "Foreword." In *Thought as Passion* by Frank Visser, xi–xv. Translated by Rachel Horner. Albany: State University of New York Press, 2003.

Williams, Florence. *The Nature Fix: Why Nature Makes us Happier, Healthier, and More Creative.* New York: W.W. Norton & Company Inc., 2017.

Wolf, Gary. "The Quantified Self." Ted Talk video, 05:04, TED@Cannes. Posted June 2010. https://www.ted.com/talks/gary_wolf_the_quantified_self/.

Yasko, Amy. *Feel Good Nutrigenomics.* Bethel, ME: Neurological Research Institute LLC, 2014.

Zhang, Yiping, and Sabine Koch. "Mobile Health Apps in Sweden: What do Physicians Recommend?" *Studies in Health Technology and Informatics, Digital Healthcare Empowering Europeans* 210 (2015): 793–797. doi: 10.3233/978-1-61499-512-8-793.

Reader Reflections

Reader Reflections

Reader Reflections

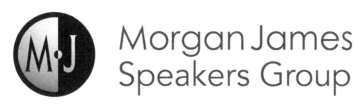

Morgan James
Speakers Group

We connect Morgan James published authors with live and online events and audiences who will benefit from their expertise.

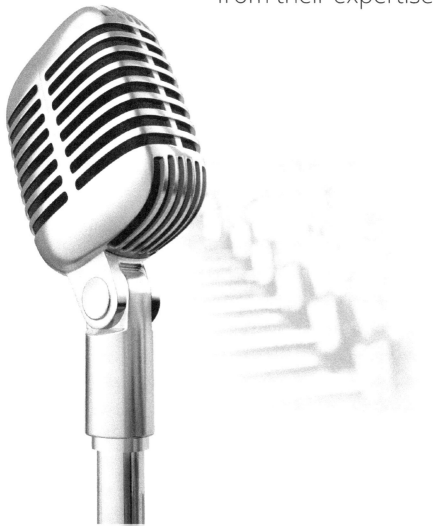

Printed in the USA
CPSIA information can be obtained
at www.ICGtesting.com
JSHW022210140824
68134JS00018B/970